The Other Side of the Bed
A Memoir

By
Andy Celella

The Other Side of the Bed
Copyright © 2023 by Andy Celella

ISBN   979-8-218-96813-7

Printed in USA

To Ralphie and Vinny

Thursday, June 20, 2019

First, the dog died. Angus, a beautiful Great Dane and Black Lab mix, weighing 100 pounds, was a selfless and kind creature. We had rescued him from a shelter after he was found in the snowy woods. He was about a year old when we got him in September 2011. He was my wife Caitlin's first dog, and our first dog together. He would break through ice just to swim and always wanted to be outside no matter the weather. He also never missed a meal. Earlier that June, he had stopped eating. A trip to the vet found he had a tick-born illness called anaplasmosis, and he was started on doxycycline antibiotics. He still was not eating and began getting weaker. We took our daily walk and he barely made it into the house. We had to bring my six-month-old son, Vinny, to the pediatrician that morning, so I told Angus, "I'll bring you to the vet when we come home."

Vinny was looking good and got his shots from the pediatrician. We grabbed some lunch at a local pizza place. We got home, brought the kids inside, and did not see Angus's usual friendly "welcome home" greeting. I went to look for him, and he was laying on our bedroom floor, prone, tongue out, and not breathing. I ran back to Caitlin and said in a hurried whisper, "Angus is FUCKING dead!"

We tried to compose ourselves, acting like everything was normal. I just shut the door so my two-and-a-half-year-old son, Ralphie, wouldn't have to see him. Caitlin read Ralphie a story and put him down for a nap while holding back tears. After he was asleep, we lifted Angus's 100 pounds of dead weight into my car, and I drove him to the vet to be cremated.

I got home and sat with Caitlin and we both cried for a couple hours while the boys slept. It was heartbreaking to lose a pet who was such a huge part of our first eight years of marriage. I called my best friend, Jeff, to tell him we couldn't have him and his two daughters over that day, as Angus had just died. Tragically enough, Jeff's mother had died one week earlier and he had sent the same text message of "sorry we can't come today." Death seemed to be lingering in the air, as my neighbor's mother had also passed about two weeks earlier. I said my customary prayer whenever I heard someone died, "May light perpetual shine upon them," (followed by a shot of whiskey this time).

We had some close friends over that evening. They had been touched by Angus's spirit and shared in our grief. We drank in memory of him. Around 9:30 PM, everyone left, and Caitlin and I headed for bed. In our bedroom lay Vinny, sleeping in his bassinet. We moved with slow, melancholy steps into bed and fell asleep.

The next thing I recall was being awakened by police and ambulance personnel in my bedroom. I heard a faint "Oh, here he comes," from one of the paramedics. I tried to sit up, but I was held down. My memory of the next few hours is spotty. It was about 11:30 PM.

Caitlin later told me that I had suffered a seizure—sat bolt upright in the dark with gagging sounds, fallen out of bed into the dead dog's bed, and had snoring respirations. Caitlin immediately called 911 and asked for no sirens, as Ralphie was still sleeping. Holding our six-month-old son, she ran over to the neighbors' and banged on the door so someone could watch the kids until my parents arrived. As the police and ambulance arrived, I was hoisted into bed and Caitlin wrestled my clothes on.

In my postictal state, I was loaded into the ambulance and brought to Yale New Haven Hospital (YNHH). Caitlin had a choice to send me to Midstate Medical Center (a Hartford Healthcare affiliate and my current employer) or to YNHH, where I had no direct coworkers. She chose YNHH so I didn't have to be seen in this condition by the doctors I worked with. Halfway to New Haven, I was looking around the ambulance and saw my old friend Cory.

"Hey Cory, what's going on?" I asked.

He looked away and said in a loud voice, "He's back, he's going to be fine."

Cory and I had worked together at Campion Ambulance Service. I also knew the other two ambulance personnel, Azeem and James (whom we called "Mojito"), from my days as an EMT. It was the first of many surreal moments I was to have on the other side of the bed, switching from provider to patient.

I was brought to YNHH ER and started on a medication called Levetiracetam (Keppra), an anti-seizure medication. I had never had a seizure before that night. I was in good health overall, except that I probably drank too much alcohol and was slightly overweight. However, I had been strong enough to run five miles earlier that morning and carry my 100-pound dog's body to the crematorium without too much effort. I had no previous medical history, no prior surgeries, and took no medications. I'd had no warning signs of the seizure. No headaches; I used to get migraines only once or twice a year, but hadn't gotten one in four years, no vision changes, no dizziness or lightheadedness. I never saw it coming.

The standard of practice for someone with a new-onset seizure is a CT scan. A Computerized Topography (CT) scan is a quick way to get information about the brain. It takes mere minutes to complete and can show severe abnormalities quickly so interventions can be started. It looks like a giant doughnut with a table extending through the doughnut hole. A patient will lay down on the table which moves through the hole, and radiation, akin to an X-ray, gives a 3D picture of whatever is scanned. The results can be seen immediately.

I was sent to a CT scanner and had my head scanned. By this time, I was completely lucid and starting to make jokes with the staff. I felt comfortable in that environment, as I have moved patients, ordered, and interpreted scans for hundreds of patients under my care. I was brought back to the ER room and waited for the results. YNHH is a teaching hospital, so I was seen by the resident who had ordered the CT scan. I heard snippets of him speaking with his attending physician.

"Oh, yep, there it is. That's a huge mass."

Casual, simple facts. Just another day at the office.

Seeing a life change right in front of you is the norm in medicine, especially ER medicine. Words I have muttered while snacking on something or drinking coffee, casual, simple: "Wow that's a big mass, probably cancer. Bummer, I have to make a bunch of calls and tell this poor bastard."

I turned to Caitlin and said, "Holy shit, I have a brain tumor."

"No, no. You don't know that. It's probably someone else," she replied.

"Yes, I know it's me. I can hear them talking about it outside the room!"

Suddenly a knock. The ER resident was a guy a few years younger than me with short blonde hair, scrubs, and a lab coat. Coffee on his breath. Sorrow on his face.

"I'm so sorry to tell you this, but it looks like you have a brain mass, and it's pretty big."

Fuck.

Shock. Mouths agape. Caitlin and I stared.

Holy shit.

When will I wake up from this nightmare?

The resident seemed quite upset telling us this. He had a wife and young kids at home; he was essentially just like me. Young guy, in good shape, medical career, wife, kids, Yale education. I think he saw himself on the stretcher where I lay. He gathered his thoughts and said the next step would be an MRI to get a better idea of what the CT scan showed.

Magnetic resonance imaging (MRI) uses magnets to create different magnetic fields to elucidate better aspects of tissue. For example, if you fall and tweak your knee, with a good amount of radiation, a CT scan can show a broken bone and if there was active hemorrhage. However, it would not be able to show if there were any tendon, ligament, or muscular abnormalities. An MRI, on the other hand, can show the bones, cartilage, tendons, ligaments, and musculature while using magnetic fields. Medical providers can use their clinical judgment to choose CT or MRI in a clinical situation based on a multitude of factors, such as cost (MRI is much more expensive than CT), if there is a contraindication (MRI cannot be used with people who have metal implants or certain pacemakers), and clinical factors (like if the CT would give the same information faster and for half the price).

In my situation, guidelines dictate that an MRI with and without contrast would give the best information to determine the next steps. The MRI could show with better efficacy what this mass was— tumor, bleeding, prediction of malignancy vs. anatomic variant. The use of a gadolinium-based contrast is used to enhance the visibility of the anatomic structures wherever the MRI is completed. So I was emergently scheduled for a brain MRI around 2 AM that Friday.

Medical Journey

My journey in the medical field was not linear. I always had a fascination with how the body works and the really divine way we are all put together. However, as a typical teenage boy who watched too many war movies growing up, I was more interested in the blood, guts, and gore. I loved watching the show "Trauma: Life in the ER," a documentary-style TV show looking at people coming into large city ERs with all the stabbings, shootings, car collisions, medical mysteries, and hilarity that humanity can offer. I was hooked. I knew I wanted to be involved in these life-or-death moments.

At 17 years old, I enrolled in an emergency medical technician (EMT) course at Hunter's Ambulance Company in Meriden, Connecticut. I learned the basics of emergency medical care for the sick and injured. I completed the course and was certified as an EMT around my 18th birthday. I started at Campion Ambulance Service in Waterbury, Connecticut. Waterbury had its heyday in the early 1800s, known for its brass manufacturing. By the time I was working there in 2006, it was home to a largely disenfranchised population of about 110,000. Within my first few weeks on the job, I had responded to car accidents, heroin overdoses, domestic violence disputes, bloody assault victims, alcohol overdoses, seizure fits, respiratory problems, strokes, and a cardiac arrest requiring CPR. I had gotten my wish; I was on the front line of these life-or-death moments. Witnessing people living and dying while in your care was such a powerful experience for an 18-year-old boy. I felt like I was in those war movies. I wanted more, and it was an honor to be able to help people at critical times in their lives.

I went to college at Northeastern University in Boston, Massachusetts. While attending classes to earn my Bachelor of Science in Health Science, I took a job at Tufts Medical Center in their ER. Located on the edge of Chinatown, the level 2 trauma center was a lesson in humanity at its worst and best. Learning how the doctors and nurses worked together to treat the sick and injured, I was an ER technician, part of the trauma response team, and essentially a jack of all trades. I would provide immediate interventions to the critically ill or injured; giving CPR was as routine as having a cup of coffee. I would coordinate set up and execution of routine interventions such as lumbar punctures, central lines, shunt placement, chest and nasogastric tube placements, and diagnostic tests such as ultrasounds, X-rays, and CT scans. Working mostly third shift, there was no shortage of crazy stories and misadventures. I loved not only the adrenaline rush but also the feeling of healing people when they were at their worst. A comforting hand or warm blanket with a friendly smile can heal more than some medications. I worked at the ER for three years during my studies at Northeastern.

Part of Northeastern University's education is the co-op program. It is a time to take a break from the classroom and work full-time in the area of your study. I went to work at the operating room at the Massachusetts Eye and Ear Infirmary. Again, a jack of all trades, my title was Operating Room Assistant. My primary responsibilities included cleaning and sanitizing operating rooms in between surgical cases as well as aseptic set up of surgical equipment, instruments, drapes, and dressings. I would handle specimen and patient transport, maintain inventory of supplies, and deliver sterile instruments and other equipment to surgeries in progress. In such a rewarding and challenging environment, I got to bump elbows with world-renowned surgeons and nurses performing numerous surgical procedures of the head, neck, face, eyes, ears, and cosmetic alterations. I worked there for the duration of my six-month co-op in 2008.

Wanting to pursue medical school training for an MD, I was essentially stonewalled by my advisors at Northeastern, as my GPA was around 3.4. Not exactly medical school material, mostly because I was working all night in the ER and would often stay awake for 36 or more hours. This wasn't conducive to maintaining a perfect GPA. I graduated from Northeastern with a B.S. in Health Sciences in May 2010. Then I left Boston and returned to my hometown in Connecticut. After a few months of odd jobs at nursing homes and some more EMT work, Caitlin and I were married in October 2011. I was actually unemployed when we got married.

To pay the bills, I started working as a phlebotomist at YNHH. A great gig for the work-life balance, with normal business hours, good pay, and benefits. I got really good at sticking needles into veins with precision and little pain, and I learned the various lab tests and why they would be used. I worked in outpatient facilities all over New Haven County. But it quickly became a bore, as it is fairly simple work; needle goes in, blood comes out, next patient. I wanted more contact with patients, more adrenaline, and more freedom to treat people the way they ought to be treated.

I quickly resigned myself to the fact that I wasn't going to medical school, mostly because of what I had been told by my advisors at Northeastern. After some reflection, I realized my philosophy of care was more akin to a nursing role than that of a doctor. I liked being at the bedside and speaking with people face-to-face, and being able to look people in the eye and give them hope—the gritty work that is nursing. So I looked toward graduate schools and found an opportunity at Yale School of Nursing (YSN). Through the Graduate Entry Pre-specialty Nursing (GEPN) program, I could get my RN license in one year and then my master's degree in two more years as an Adult/Gerontology Acute Care Nurse Practitioner. I was accepted into the program and started in August 2012.

While studying at Yale, I continued to work per diem as a phlebotomist. YSN was a challenging and rewarding three years. I don't think I have ever worked so hard to succeed as I did through that rigorous program. In a cohort of 80 students, we all had different backgrounds and survived a twelve-month blitzkrieg in nursing practice. Given my variety of medical experience, I fared quite well and managed to pass the NCLEX in September 2013, becoming a Registered Nurse. I worked that year at the Yale Health Plan, treating Yale students, faculty, and staff who were all on the Yale Health Plan.

I then started on the master's degree portion of the curriculum under the director, Dr. Laura Andrews. She was a fierce leader and would teach with profanity and kindness, truly an awe-inspiring presence. We had a heavy course load coupled with an arduous clinical assignment. My specialty was acute care and mostly ICU care. I spent most of my clinical hours in the medical ICU at the Hospital of Central Connecticut, under the direction of Dr. Steven Prunk. I was welcomed into the group of blurry-eyed medical residents. I spent five months with about 40 hours per week in that ICU, spending more time in the ICU than most internal medicine doctors do throughout their residencies. I worked just like the medical residents; I managed care, developed treatment plans, and wrote progress/transfer notes for patients in the ICU, plus gave presentations for our attending physicians. I learned how to respond to medical emergencies such as septic shock, rhabdomyolysis, ischemic/hemorrhagic stroke, severe ETOH withdrawal, hypoxic/hypercapnic respiratory failure, DIC, ARDS, and multisystem organ dysfunction. I completed several procedures, including: central line insertions, arterial line insertions, arterial blood gas collections, and NG feeding tube placements. By the time I finished my rotation, I had won the respect of medical residents and attending physicians and learned so much about care for the hospitalized patient.

In addition to the medical ICU training, Yale School of Nursing gave me the opportunity to complete rotations in the Hartford Hospital Cardiothoracic ICU. I managed care for patients who'd had any sort of open-heart surgeries, such as: coronary artery bypass grafts (CABGs), ventricular assist devices (L/R VADs), balloon pumps, Impella pumps, transcatheter aortic valve replacements (TAVRs), aortic dissection repairs, and cardiac tamponade. I also completed procedures such as arterial line insertions, Swan Ganz catheter placements, and observed LVAD placement in the OR. Suffice it to say I happily did it all.

My final rotation at Yale was a Hospitalist Service rotation at YNHH. I managed care and developed treatment plans for inpatients admitted under the hospitalist service. I completed physical exams, wrote progress notes, coordinated care between specialties, completed medication reconciliation, arranged for follow up appointments, and assisted in discharge planning. This view of general medicine and managing care appealed to me, as each day was always so different, and there was always something new to learn.

Upon my graduation from Yale School of Nursing with a Master's of Nursing in May 2015, I felt well prepared for my future medical career. I took a job at Bristol Hospital as a hospitalist in November 2015. I was working a 7-on 7-off shift, which meant I would work seven days (Monday-Sunday) and then have the next week off. Located in a small community hospital with 150 beds serving a city of 60,000 and the surrounding area, the hospitalist position was quite an introduction to hospital medicine. In the first week, I pronounced three people dead, told two they had cancer, and another that he had full-blown AIDS. The community had many blue-collar workers with poor health habits, like smoking, alcohol and drug use, diabetes, and generally not taking care of themselves. Often patients would come into the hospital with some problem, had not seen a doctor in 30 or 40 years, and would be promptly diagnosed with some horrible disease or cancer. Many difficult patients, but also many lovely, kind people who just wanted another chance at health and would follow "doctor's orders" well.

I spent three years at Bristol Hospital, working almost 90 hours one week and then zero hours the next. The small community of doctors and nurses was truly a friendly, loving, supportive, and generous family to me. When I first started, I was absolutely terrified to take care of patients all by myself. My "orientation" was seeing six patients the first day, ten patients the next, and then an average of 15-20 daily after that. This is in stark contrast to some of my fellow Yale grads, who spent 6-9 months on orientation, or doctors who spend three years in residency. I was the only nurse practitioner on the hospitalist team, and I found such great mentorship and support in all my fellow doctor/hospitalists and specialists. Within a few months, I was taking 15-20 patients during the morning, two or three admissions per day, answering cross-coverage calls for the entire hospital (including ICU patients), and going to every rapid response call for patients requiring immediate attention.

The whole hospitalist group was employed by a contracting company called Team Health. The Bristol Hospital leadership decided not to renew the contract with Team Health beginning January 2019. The company that replaced Team Health offered me a $15,000 pay cut, so I began looking for a new job.

I was given a fantastic and generous package with Hartford Healthcare, where I continued in a hospitalist role, but worked only Saturday, Sunday, and Monday each week. I was working fewer hours, getting paid more, and given advancement opportunities and more time with my family. This was especially important, since my second son was born two weeks before I started the position on December 31, 2018. I was on top of the world, and everything was going great until I was kicked to the other side of the hospital bed.

Friday, June 21, 2019

In the wee hours of that Friday morning, I was moved from my small room in the Yale ER to the MRI department, down a long dimly lit hallway. Trepidation and fear started to creep in during the cold stretcher ride. I began to think of the worst possible thing that could appear on the MRI.

Medical practitioners are taught to form a differential diagnosis. Essentially, one looks at a clinical problem and thinks of all the possible causes of the problem. Then the practitioner thinks of the causes that would kill the patient the fastest and rules those things out. For instance, if you go to the ER with chest pain, the first thing is to make sure you're not having a serious problem which needs immediate fixing or intervention. So you may get an EKG to make sure the heart rhythm is ok. Then you may get a chest X-ray to see if there is any major lung problem (like a collapsed lung) or if any big artery is bleeding (aortic aneurysm rupture). If you were having a heart attack (seen on EKG), a lung collapse (found on chest X-ray), or severe bleeding (seen on chest X-ray or CT scan), immediate action would need to be taken so that you could stay alive. A good practitioner will ask you the right questions and conduct an accurate history and physical to help make the correct diagnosis, which is why you get asked the same questions by everyone at the hospital.

When a medical provider looks at a new onset unprovoked seizure, the current literature gives the following differential: syncope (fainting with some confusion or convulsion), transient ischemic attack (mini-stroke), migraines, panic attack and anxiety, psychogenic nonepileptic seizure (fainting for some reason, but not epilepsy), transient global amnesia (sudden forgetfulness), narcolepsy with cataplexy, paroxysmal movement disorders, cardiac arrhythmia, vasovagal syncope, metabolic conditions (such as electrolyte abnormalities), vascular conditions (i.e., transient ischemic attacks).

Wow, what a list.

That list is really only a fraction of what the average provider is thinking when ordering the next test to start ruling out some of those conditions and narrowing down the cause of the seizure. Again, the general idea is to rule out the thing that will kill you first, and then work from there. So as a nurse practitioner who routinely worked in hospital and ICU medical care with a background in ER medicine, I had a hard time escaping from that way of thinking. I was always thinking of the worst possible thing that could happen so that I could fix it. It is terrifying to think about the worst-case scenario in terms of your own brain as you are wheeled down to the next test.

I arrived at the MRI department and was stripped of my clothes, watch, wedding ring, jewelry, and other metallic items. It was the first of many times I would feel completely exposed and naked around strangers, feelings I rarely considered while providing care to patients. I was then awed by the many MRIs I'd ordered without thinking about all the patients would endure to get the procedure done. I was placed on the MRI table with a blanket, as I was shivering in the cold room. I was given ear plugs and a large plastic plate was attached to the table, only a few inches from my face. As I was moved into position to enter a bigger and louder doughnut, I closed my eyes.

The brain MRI with and without contrast takes 30-45 minutes to complete. The first 15-25 minutes are marked by the banging and mild shaking of the machine. This first phase gives the non-contrast pictures. Then the table moves out and a technician comes in to inject the contrast. A gadolinium-based contrast was administered through my IV. Fortunately, I had no allergic reactions. Some people can feel the contrast flowing through them or have certain sensations associated with it, like the taste of metal. I had a little taste of metal, but it quickly subsided. The remainder of the test is completed with the same clinks, bangs, and table movements. After about 45 minutes, I was brought back to the waiting area to retrieve my clothes, watch, jewelry, and ring. I was wheeled by stretcher back to the emergency department.

I was slated to be admitted to the hospital. Unfortunately, I was also supposed to work that morning at the Hospital of Central Connecticut (HOCC), a sister hospital of Midstate Medical Center. My former boss from Bristol Hospital, Dr. Adiraju, had given me a few shifts to get on board with HOCC and have some added shifts and income. I called her at 3 AM to let her know I wasn't coming in to work. She called me back a few minutes later and was horrified at the news. This was the first person I had called with the news, and

I will always remember the words that came out of my mouth: staid, yet so surreal.

Waiting in the ER for a bed in the hospital is akin to having a flight permanently on standby. You are buckled into your seat but cannot move because the seatbelt sign is on. You are told by the captain that, "There are a few planes ahead of us, and we'll get clearance from the tower soon." You wait and wait. No way to move, no getting up, no peanuts, no drinks, yet more waiting. The ER feels the same way. Every once in a while, different hospital staff will pop in to ask you a few questions, like insurance information, next of kin, or emergency contacts, but will offer no information on when you will be moved or how far along the process is. It often seems like no one knows anything about your case. They are concerned about getting their questions answered, not answering yours. As you sit there waiting, you hear different people around your room speaking softly about what infection they have, and what the doctors want to do about it. Sometimes there is moaning, screaming, fits of anger. It is how I imagine purgatory, the land between heaven and hell.

If you are admitted to the hospital, a cascade of events needs to occur. First, the ER doctor will determine if you need to be admitted to the hospital. Then they will ask one of the hospital's services to place the admission orders. The admission orders initiate teams of people to find a bed, then manage financial aspects and insurance claims. This service is typically a group of physicians in a certain specialty, such as the surgery service (if you need surgery), or cardiology service (if you were having a heart attack), or the hospitalist service (general internal medicine). One particular service will usually see and examine you in the ER, and agree to admit you under their attending physician. That attending physician is responsible for overseeing your time in the hospital. Different services may be consulted about your care. For example, you may be admitted under the hospitalist service if you have a serious infection; the hospitalist may then call an infectious disease specialist to give their expert opinion on your care, like before giving medication to treat your infection. Then the hospitalist, or primary attending, will follow the consultants' advice, and when the patient is well enough, they are discharged from the hospital.

As we were waiting in the ER, my father arrived with some coffee and breakfast. I had a cup of coffee and stared blankly out into the hallway. Around 9 AM, there was a knock at the door. I looked up out of my trance and saw a pretty brunette woman in her late 30s standing in the doorway. She introduced herself as Dr. Jennifer Moliterno from the Neurosurgery team. She was to be the brain surgeon who would be admitting me and performing brain surgery. She pulled up the images from the MRI and explained that there was a large mass, likely a low-grade glioma, measuring 3.6 cm x 2.5 cm x 3.6 cm, about the size of a golf ball. A glioma is a tumor which may or may not be malignant. Its name refers to glial cells which make up brain tissue. She pointed out the tumor on the computer screen. It was located above my left ear, known as the left temporal lobe, in the part of the brain known as Wernicke area. The Wernicke area is the primary area responsible for language. Dr. Moliterno explained that I would need brain surgery to remove as much of the tumor as possible. Because the tumor was in the language and speech area of the brain, I would have to be awake during the surgery so they could monitor my speech while they were removing the golf ball-sized tumor.

"You will stay in the hospital over the weekend, get pre-op testing on Monday, and we'll do surgery on Tuesday. Any questions?" Dr. Moliterno asked sweetly.

Holy FUCK!

Yes, thousands of questions! Let me get this straight: I have a golf ball in my brain, so you're essentially going to stick knives and a melon baller into my BRAIN, and take out the tumor while I'm AWAKE? ARE YOU FUCKING SERIOUS?

"No questions," I said while nodding like an idiot, trying to absorb the information.

"Great! See you later," she said warmly. She hugged my sobbing wife and left.

Caitlin was sitting crying in the corner of the room, and my father had his mouth agape. Since I had the medical training, my family looked to me for answers and more importantly, translation of medical treatments and procedures. After hearing what my plan of care was going to be, I was speechless.

My head was still spinning from hearing the news about my brain tumor and the plan to have an awake craniotomy. I began to furiously research my condition. I found conditions of different types of gliomas. I looked up information on awake craniotomies. Caitlin and my father kept vigil with me, leaving only for coffee or to go back and forth to visit our kids at home. My mother and grandmother were watching the kids at my house and keeping everyone busy. At one point, my family had left and I was dozing off in the ER, when a tall, staid German man entered. He introduced himself as Dr. Baehring from Neuro-Oncology. He stated he would continue to follow my case and see me after surgery. He would make arrangements to follow up in his office after biopsy and surgical reports. It was a very quick meeting, as there was limited information at this point. I took his card and promptly dozed off again. Little did I know that over the next few months I would come to despise, then truly admire, become grateful for, and ultimately indebted to Dr. Baehring.

That afternoon, after about 36 hours in the ER, I was moved up to East Pavilion 7-7 on the seventh floor of YNHH. I was admitted to the Neurosurgery service under Dr. Moliterno. Fortunately, I was given a private room with a shower and bathroom. Since I had been a YNHH employee as a phlebotomist, attended Yale Nursing School, and completed several clinical rotations throughout YNHH, they treated me like one of their own. I was able to view my lab reports, progress notes, CT/MRI results, and other documentation. I was cleared to come and go as I pleased. I did not need to call someone to help me to the bathroom, nor was I receiving intensive care; I was there for pre-op and to receive one pill in the morning and one pill at night—both Keppra, my anti-seizure regimen. I was very friendly to everyone and a floor nurse's best patient—no dumb questions nor stupid requests, and functioning completely independently.

I took the freedom quite liberally. I walked all over the hospital while other patients with my same condition would have been on bed rest with seizure precautions. I was walking around the hospital with a Yale sweatshirt and shorts, my IV and hospital band tucked underneath, acting like I was there on hospital/school business. If I had suffered another seizure, there would have been hell to pay for my nurses, doctors, my East Pavilion floor, and YNHH in general. If I was the hospitalist attending and saw one of my patients doing what I was doing, I would be furious. I lived up to the well-known statement: doctors make the worst patients. In retrospect, I was actually quite reckless.

The weekend continued in the same fancy-free fashion, albeit with some business first. Each day, I was woken by the phlebotomist around 4 AM with bright light streaming into my eyes and sharp needles probing my veins. The neurosurgery resident would arrive around 5 AM to do a quick exam, make sure I wasn't having any seizures, and then reiterate the plan for preoperative exams on Monday, followed by surgery on Tuesday. I would doze groggily until about 7 AM, when I would order my breakfast and meet the oncoming nurse for the day. I got my morning pill, 1000 milligrams of Levetiracetam (Keppra), by 9 AM. Then I was seen by the neurology surgery fellow, covering for the neuro-oncology service. There were a resident and attending who would enter, do a quick exam, and reiterate the plan for the weekend, surgery, and follow up with Dr. Baehring.

After the residents saw me, they would return with their attending providers to again review the plans. This is standard practice for most teaching hospitals. It can be very frustrating for patients to have to repeat the same conversations and get different answers from the attendings, but that's how doctors and other providers learn to care for their patients. I was very accustomed to seeing the residents, as I had worked with so many during my training and had been a teacher for PAs and APRNs. I would often quiz the residents or ask them questions about their presentations of my case. The residents became a nuisance to Caitlin, but they provided an opportunity for me to gain some control of my circumstance and feel like I was back on the other side of the bed, in my lab coat with my students discussing a patient's plan of care.

After the morning visits were over, I would start my walking. I knew the hospital so well because I had spent so many years as an employee and student at Yale. I knew where the best and cleanest bathrooms were. I knew where the quiet places were. I spent a lot of time in the hospital chapel and the Healing Garden, a Zen-like rooftop garden on the seventh floor of Smilow Cancer Hospital. Some of my favorite places to reflect on patients I'd had as a student now served as my refuge, a space to sort out my own thoughts. I thought of my own mortality and my family. I vacillated between patient and provider. I would recall my blood work, vital signs, notes, imaging, and think of my own clinical picture and how I would manage a patient like me.

Caitlin and other family and friends would visit at different times during the day. Often I was on a walk while someone came to my room, and they would call me so I could meet them back at my room. On day one of my inpatient stay, my mother-in-law Colleen called and asked how we were doing since Angus's passing.

"Oh, we are well beyond that, and things are much worse now," replied Caitlin.

On Sunday, even more of my family from out of state came to visit. Caitlin brought the kids and we hung out in the first-floor lobby, where there were lots of plants and huge water fountain features. The kids ran and played as if they were at a Sunday BBQ. Us adults spoke in hushed tones as I explained the plan for the brain surgery. I slipped into medical jargon while speaking with my uncles, who are cardiologists and ophthalmologists. It was a surreal time, as I was still in good health, yet here we were in the hospital, a golf ball invading my head, with my kids running and playing. As the evening drew to a close, everyone said their goodbyes and I returned to my room. I had a restless night, as I was preparing myself for pre-operative testing the following day.

Medical Hierarchy

It is worth describing the general hierarchy of hospital staff for those who are not in the industry. Medical Assistants (MA)—also known as Patient Care Associates (PCA), Patient Care Technicians (PCT), or Certified Nursing Assistants (CNA), depending on the hospital—are the people who help the nursing staff with general patient care. They provide vital sign measurements, assist in activities of daily living (ADLs) such as toileting, changing clothing/bedding, phlebotomy, and are usually the first people to come if you press the call bell in the hospital. The MAs usually have at least an associate's degree or have completed additional coursework to earn a certification.

Registered Nurses (RN) are the people that deliver the care with the MAs. They are the ones that give you your medications and other interventions. There is a huge variety of RN responsibilities depending on where the RN is working. On the neurology floor, they were responsible for giving medications, monitoring neurological changes and mental status, and assisting the doctors in any procedures. The RN at your primary care provider's office may have a very different responsibility. The RN degree is completed after an associate's or bachelor's degree and is contingent on passing the licensing board's National Council Licensure Examination-RN (NCLEX-RN).

Physician Associates (PA) and Nurse Practitioners (NP or APRN) are known collectively as Advanced Practice Providers (APP). A

PA will have a four-year undergraduate degree, and then a three-year graduate degree. Specific residencies are available in some places, but more common is on-the-job training in a given area. PAs work under and are supervised by MDs. APRNs will have a four-year undergraduate degree, hold an RN license, and then a two- or three-year graduate degree, and may hold additional degrees such as Doctor of Nursing Practice (DNP). Depending on the state, APRNs can work under an MD license, practice in collaboration, or practice independently. In Connecticut, I am an Adult/Gerontology Acute Care Nurse Practitioner (AGACNP), board-certified, and practice independently. My specialty is acute care/critical care hospital medicine. So I am a nurse with additional education, holding essentially the same credentials as a board-certified internal medicine physician.

The doctors are less straightforward. After graduating with an undergraduate degree, a person applies to medical school. Once admitted, the aspiring doctor will study for four years and graduate with a Medical Doctorate (MD). After graduating from the fourth year of medical school, the student is now called a doctor. During the middle of March in the fourth year of medical school, there is Match Day. Match Day is when the fourth-year medical student is accepted into a residency program. There are different specialties that start at this stage. Internal medicine, surgery, neurosurgery, anesthesiology, and emergency medicine start here. Residencies begin on July 1st every year. The first year is called the intern year, followed by two more years (depending on the specialty) to then be ready for board certification. After about three years (again, depending on the specialty) and board certification, the resident becomes an attending physician.

Specialist physicians have additional education time. After an internal medicine residency of three years, the doctor may choose to pursue a fellowship in a certain specialty. Cardiologists, gastroenterologists, infectious disease specialists, neurologists, and pulmonologists enter another three to eight years of fellowship study before they are board certified.

Let's look at my team for an example of the amount of schooling one doctor had completed. Neurosurgeon Dr. Moliterno attended four years of undergrad, four years of medical school, one year of residency at Yale, followed by six to eight years of neurosurgery residency, a chief residency, and then an additional one-year clinical fellowship in neurosurgical oncology specializing in surgery for brain and spinal cord tumors at the Memorial Sloan-Kettering Cancer Center in New York City. Altogether, she had 18 years of neurosurgery training prior to her board certification. That is a long time to spend in education, but I'm glad people who are digging around in the brain have such thorough training.

Monday, June 24, 2019

Monday morning started like the other mornings on the seventh floor—a 4 AM blood draw. But this time, more vials were taken in order to check my blood type, how fast my blood would clot, and my liver and kidney functions. Then the neurosurgery resident arrived around 5 AM. She outlined my schedule for the day. First, blood work, which had just been collected. Then I was to have a chest X-ray to ensure there were no obvious lung issues. A functional MRI around 8 AM. The team would review the results of all the tests and see me again later that afternoon, when consent for the surgery would be completed. I agreed, and she left.

I took my morning Keppra and had a small breakfast. Around 7:30 AM, a portly man came with a stretcher to wheel me down to the MRI suite. I removed all my clothing and metallic objects and put on a hospital gown. I was wanded to ensure I didn't have any metallic items and brought into the MRI scanner.

The functional MRI (FMRI) is different than a conventional MRI. Developed by a Japanese researcher, Seiji Ogawa, in 1990, the relatively new technology is used more for research than in a clinical/medical setting. The FMRI typically uses a blood-oxygen-level dependent contrast that lights up areas of the brain. The FMRI would detect different areas of the brain to show where my cognition and especially speech were originating. It was a longer MRI (approximately 60 minutes), and I had to look at a screen on which words would appear while I lay supine in the MRI. These words ranged from simple words such as "banana" or "coffee" to more complex words such as "euphoric" or "malaise." Alongside these words were plus or minus signs. I was instructed to focus on the plus or minus sign and think about the word that was on the screen. I did not speak throughout the MRI; I merely had to think about the words, and this would cause different areas of my brain to light up. This gives a unique picture which shows exactly where the areas essential to my cognition were located. This information was paired with the original MRI scan and provided Dr. Moliterno with additional information prior to and during the brain surgery.

After the test, I was brought back to my room. Dr. Moliterno and her team saw me later that morning. The procedure was again outlined for me, and it was to begin early the next morning. I was then given a consent form. In every surgical case, the patient needs to be informed of all possible risks, benefits, and alternatives for the surgery. When I read the form, I couldn't help but focus on the horrible things that could happen during the surgical procedure, including but not limited to: blood loss and need for blood transfusion, permanent brain damage, stroke, heart attack, incomplete tumor removal, and of course, death.

Holy shit.

Ok. I guess I have no real alternative, and hopefully all goes well.

I signed the form and said "I'll see you all tomorrow."

While anxiously pondering the consent form I had just signed, I was then visited by a woman who introduced herself as Jenn Bernstein of Fox 61 News, a local news station based in Hartford, Connecticut. She wanted to film my brain surgery because I would be awake and talking. Apparently, this usually grabs a few extra viewers and makes for a good news story. She asked permission to film the surgery and put it on the evening news. She offered me a consent form. There was nothing about "blood loss, stroke, brain damage, or death," so I signed it, thinking that it was nowhere near as bad as the form I had signed earlier. Their consent form seemed quite unremarkable.

I remember an odd mixture of feelings—mostly bliss and sadness—at the end of this day. It felt like I was preparing for a great battle. I showered and shaved in the hospital bathroom while looking in the mirror. I was wondering if this was going to be the last day I would see myself in a mirror. I looked down and cringed at the nature of the crude hospital shower setting.

So many questions: Would I see my wife and kids again? Would I be alive at the end of the day tomorrow? Would I retain my brain function and get back to my life and work? Would I wake up with a British accent and have no recollection of my past life? Would I gain a superpower like some cheesy comic book?

Despite the trepidation, I slept surprisingly well and was ready for surgery the next day.

Tuesday, June 25, 2019

Pre-op

I awoke early the next morning. The neurosurgery team rounded at 5 AM. Caitlin had stayed the night in case that was the last time she would see me. I was ready for battle. I was wheeled down to the pre-op area around 7:30. My stomach growled, as I couldn't have anything to eat or drink prior to the surgery. I was placed in a holding station near the OR. There were several stretchers around the large room with a central nurse's station. A flurry of OR staff in gray and pink scrubs moved around the room like a huge beehive. I was accompanied by my father and Caitlin.

Dr. Moliterno visited and gave Caitlin a hug as she cried softly. "Everything will go well. I guess you really like him," she said to Caitlin. She turned to me and asked how I was feeling.

"I'm feeling good. I'm ready for this." She smiled kindly and gave other assurances, then disappeared through the OR doors.

Then there was a line of people who needed to talk with me. We met an OR nurse named Ingrid; our lifelong friend, Linda, had told us to look for her as an inside source of information. Ingrid gave Caitlin and my father her personal cell phone number and offered to keep in communication with them throughout the surgery. Then we met Paul, my circulation RN. His job was to promote teamwork, coordinate supplies, and keep open communication with the surgeons and other OR staff. Circulation RNs are not "scrubbed in," meaning they do not put on all the extra surgically sterile garb worn by the surgeons, scrub technicians, and scrub nurses (the folks that were actually hovering over the open chasm of my brain).

Then the Fox 61 news crew came in. They introduced themselves and said they would take video and basically stay out of the way of the surgeons. There was a camera operator, the news anchor, Jenn, and another IT guy. The cameraman and IT guy went to set up in the OR. Jenn stayed to see the rest of the pre-op preparations.

Neurophysiologist Brooke Callahan was the next member of the OR team I met. She would be with me while I was awake during the surgery. In order to avoid cutting any vital fibers which control my speech/language, an awake craniotomy would be performed so they could monitor my speech throughout the procedure. Brooke had five to ten pages of different questions. She first asked me to say the alphabet and count from 1 to 10, listening closely for my accent and other pronunciation minutiae. She asked my name and birthday, then wrote down my answers. Then came simple open-ended questions, such as what do you put on pizza (pepperoni, cheese, sauce), and sentences I needed to finish. The weather in the winter is (cold). I stated the days of the week, months of the year.

I then mentioned that I sing with a graduate and professional choir and asked if I could sing during the surgery. I sang a short passage of Ralph Vaughan Williams' piece "Dona Nobis Pacem." The section is called "Reconciliation," and is set to a poem by Walt Whitman, who was a nurse who cared for both Northern and

Southern troops in the Civil War. The lyrics include *"Word over all, beautiful as the sky! Beautiful that war, and all its deeds of carnage, must in/time be utterly lost; That the hands of the sisters Death and Night, incessantly/softly wash again, and ever again, this soil'd world...."* I received an applause from those in the area. Jenn and the news crew's eyes lit up. They were excited to have another aspect to their news report; not only would I have my brain sliced open while awake, but now I would also sing during it! This was television gold!

The anesthesia team was next in line. They told me the procedure for how they would anesthetize me, using a medication called Propofol. It is a drug that is used in most surgeries and makes patients fall asleep rapidly, but has a very short half-life, meaning its effects diminish quickly. After the surgical team sawed through my skull and my brain and tumor were exposed, they would stop the Propofol and I would slowly wake up. Once I was awake, Dr. Moliterno and her team would start removal of the tumor. After they got as much tumor as they could, the anesthesia team would restart the Propofol, my skull would be replaced, and my scalp stapled shut. I would have another MRI in the OR to see how much of the tumor they had removed. Then I would be slowly awakened and sent to the neurosurgery ICU.

"Easy-peasy," I said.

Caitlin was not amused, again in tears. I was fairly relaxed. I had faith in the team. I had faith in God. I also figured if I died, at least

Caitlin would get my life insurance. If I was permanently brain damaged, whelp, hopefully I wouldn't even realize it. Either way, I was going into this surgery. I had no other choice but to be calm. I braced for impact like I was getting ready for the beaches of Normandy, kissed my wife goodbye, and was slowly wheeled down to the OR.

Surgery

I was positioned on the OR table. I thought, "Thank God it's not July and I don't have to worry about some dumbass intern messing me up." (First-year interns always start July 1st). I was placed supine on the operating table, leaning onto my right side to give access to the tumor on the left side of my head. I was comfortable, and I said aloud to the OR, "I'll see you all on the flip side." With that, I fell asleep and the surgery began.

My recollection of the surgery itself is quite vague. In writing this part of my story, I relied heavily on the uncut video that the news cameras filmed. Until I watched the footage, I had only remembered a few moments of the surgery; then I recalled the pain and other details.

I suddenly awoke and remembered having a pounding headache, the neurophysiologist and anesthesiologist above me. It felt as though I had woken from a very deep sleep. As I started to move my eyes around, I noticed the OR and began to appreciate my surroundings. The video showed that I would drift off, but then be shaken awake and stammer, "Yeah…yeah...sorry, I'm awake."

I only remember answering a few of the questions. I remember reciting my birthday, the days of the week, and filling in the blank to a question about what the weather is like in winter, to which I responded, "Shitty!" This was followed by the OR staff's laughter. My head hurt quite a bit. It was a sharp, burning, gnawing pain directly where the surgeon was operating. I humorously remarked "I'm not sure if it's because of the brain surgery or because I didn't have a cup of coffee this morning."

Usually quite jovial with my medical colleagues, my time under the knife was no exception. I was able to focus and keep my anxiety at bay. I answered the questions and tried to be the best patient I could, thinking that if I had to cut someone's brain open, I'd want them to be calm and confident in my ability. I remained calm and kept making bad jokes about medicine, coffee, and winter weather. My use of profanity was quite profound, and I remember apologizing by saying "I hear people with high intelligence use profanity more often…although I use this excuse when I get in trouble for using too much profanity."

To take a break from my rampant swearing, I sang the same Vaughn Williams excerpt that I had sung earlier in pre-op. It was good enough, and I received applause from the OR staff. As you can imagine, having a bunch of scalpels and scissors in your brain is not the most conducive for singing. My fellow choir members, every voice teacher I've ever had, and anyone who has a sense of pitch, would notice my severely flat tone and scooping of notes (an absolute "no-no" for the classically trained). Nevertheless, I sang (fairly well), while having the golf ball removed from my brain. Even Pavarotti can't top that!

Throughout the surgery, there were continued checks on my mental status and assurances that my speech and language stayed intact.

One indication of cutting too much of these delicate nerve fibers would be a sense of confusion or interruption in my speech pattern. At one point, they asked "What do you do with a chair?" I stuttered and answered frankly "I don't know." The neurophysiologist alerted Dr. Moliterno that the area she was cutting was causing my confusion. She would stop cutting this area and work on a different portion of my brain. Similar instances like this would occur quite often. At one point I was asked, "What do you put on pizza?" I slowly answered, "Chocolate, bananas, and ice cream."

Dr. Moliterno delicately removed as much tumor as she could without me continuing to miss words and incorrectly answer questions. About three hours into the surgery, she decided she could not remove any more. She told me that she was done and that I had done a great job. I laughed and said, "You did a good job, too! I could see the whole thing." I had been positioned with a clear view of the operating room TV screen. On this screen, which had an enlarged HD camera right on my brain, I could actually see the real-time footage of scalpels resecting the tumor in my brain. It is truly fascinating to see your own brain getting sliced and suctioned (if one has the stomach for it). I said, "Watching you cut open my brain is something I will never forget." They profusely apologized. They'd had no idea that I could see the surgery while I was awake and answering questions! I remarked "I'm pretty sure not many patients would be able to see that."

At the end of nearly two hours, I was restarted on anesthesia and drifted back into sleep. The piece of my skull was replaced with two titanium plates, and my scalp stapled closed. I was brought to an intraoperative MRI machine. The MRI showed almost 96% of the tumor had been removed.

The next thing I remember was waking up to see my wife, dressed in a Tyvek suit used by OR personnel. She had been smuggled in by one of the nurses. I told her I felt okay and everything was good. The only people left in the OR were two anesthesiology residents. I was not moved to the Post Anesthesia Care Unit (PACU) because there were no beds available. I had to wait until an ICU room was ready for me to be transferred.

Post-op

I arrived at the neurology ICU in stable condition. The absolute worst part of the surgery was the removal of my Foley catheter (which was placed while under anesthesia). Having that tube yanked from my urethra was, by far, the worst part of the surgery. I pissed what seemed like razor blades for 24 hours and actual blood for about 12 hours after the removal. It still makes me shudder as I write this.

I was offered food, although I wasn't hungry. I had some awful hospital chocolate ice cream and water. I still had a very bad headache. I had received fentanyl during the operation, but no other pain medication. I reasoned the pain was probably normal after brain surgery. I was given 1000 milligrams of Tylenol, and then my headache subsided partially. That was the last time I received any pain medication after my surgery.

My wife and my father stayed until about 6 PM. I grabbed my cell phone and attempted to read the text messages I had received. However, I could not understand any of the writing in the messages. Dumbfounded. I was able to see the words perfectly, but the words on the page just seemed not to fit together to make a coherent sentence. I assumed it was part of the surgery and anesthesia, and put the phone down. I slept well that evening and awoke early the next morning.

Wednesday, June 26, 2019

In the morning, I was barely able to read the breakfast menu. It was a very slow process to read each word then read them all again to process what the sentence said. I was akin to a first grader attempting his first Dr. Seuss book. In my brain I saw: The...words...on...the...page...don't, wait, didn't...find, wait, fit...together...Ok, "The words on the page didn't fit together." *Ok, I get it, next sentence.* It would take almost three minutes per sentence.

Anxiety cascaded through me as I discovered that I could not read. This terrifying wave of horror that I could barely understand any piece of paper presented to me. Running through my mind were thoughts of *How will I be able to return to work?*

How will I be able to read to my children?

How can I even function in an adult society so dependent on text?

I tried not to think about it too much, and blamed it on the surgery or anesthesia. At the time, I did not realize that this side effect would be much more profound and last much longer than I originally expected.

While trying to get the thought of not being able to read for the rest of my life out of my head, I began ambulating around the neurology ICU. I still had a headache; however, I was feeling good and otherwise had no further postoperative complications. I stayed in the neurology ICU for approximately 18 hours. My transfer paperwork was completed early in the morning after rounding with the neurosurgery team at 5 AM. There were no available beds on the general medical floors, so it was around 2 PM when I was transferred to East Pavilion seventh floor, the same unit I was on prior to surgery.

When I arrived on that floor, I was put into a double room. I was ambulating without difficulty, had no bed restrictions, no seizures, and I could complete all my ADLs without issue. The man next to me in my room was not as well off. He was in his late 70s, frail, and appeared older than his age. I overheard him say to his visiting family that he had been admitted with worsening confusion and was found to have a large tumor on his brain, closer to the frontal aspect. Dr. Moliterno and the neurosurgical team saw and evaluated him and would also attempt surgery within a few days.

The striking dissonance in our small hospital room echoed between the thin curtains that separated our beds. This man seemed to have several comorbidities, including some level of dementia; he was frail and barely able to get out of bed with maximum assistance. I felt my heart ache as I thought surely his prognosis was quite poor. This was in stark contrast to my young, strong body with no previous problems. I was able to get up and take a piss when I wanted, but he would struggle to find the call bell and could only mutter a faint cry for help with a bedside urinal.

I saw Dr. Baehring and his team later that afternoon, and we planned a follow up visit. At this point, I was still confident that I had a low-grade glioma and it was unlikely that I would need any further treatments. Dr. Baehring did not give me any indication either way. We would have to await biopsy studies, DNA analysis, and identification of tumor markers. It was a quick visit with the tall, serious German physician.

Dr. Moliterno and her team saw me again later that afternoon. All my blood work looked good, and I was doing well. We agreed to anticipate discharge from the hospital the following day with follow up in three weeks to remove the 38 staples that had been placed in my scalp. The operation was a success, and she was very pleased to report that 96% of the tumor had been removed. Thankfully, Dr. Moliterno is a kind and compassionate Italian woman who would give hugs freely with a warmth that penetrated deeply and resounded with, "Everything is OK."

Her team stated that as long as everything continued to make good progress, I would need to complete a few things prior to discharge. One of which was to work with the physical therapy staff to determine if I needed any services at home or if I would need an inpatient rehabilitation stay. I immediately scoffed at the idea, as I had been walking around the ICU and inpatient floor for the last day-and-a-half.

I also had to be maintained on an IV infusion of 3% saline, also known as hypertonic saline. The blood that courses through your veins and arteries has a salt content of 0.9%. In the neurosurgery setting, the hypertonic saline is used to keep sodium levels higher to improve excretion of urine and to reduce swelling in the brain. I had a 20 gauge IV in my right forearm where the hypertonic saline was running. This also can give a burning sensation; think "salt in an open wound," only in your veins.

Although I was not walking around the hospital or outside the building, I was still able to move about as I pleased. The nursing staff was excellent and would allow me to view my MRI scans and blood work, also granting me access to the progress notes of the various providers who were following me. A rare gift for any patient, and fortunately I had the knowledge and skill to interpret my medical chart. However, it would take me considerably longer to read the progress notes than it would to review MRIs and blood work.

I had a restless night, as my roommate was unable to completely move or toilet himself without assistance. He needed to call to be brought to the bathroom and for additional pain relief. I was sure he had some other comorbidities and other medical problems. He would call out at random, and given the thin curtain between us, I would awaken every time his light would turn on.

As a hospitalist, I know that the first thing a patient usually complains about is their roommate. At work, I simply apologize, knowing that I can't do anything like offer a private room or change a bed assignment. Just one night spent next to this poor soul was enough to conjure memories of everyone to whom I had curtly acknowledged or scoffed at after their complaint of a lousy neighbor. I spent years hearing these complaints, even having patients sign out of the hospital against medical advice. Now I understood why.

Thursday, June 27, 2019

Discharge day. Oh, sweet discharge day. I felt enormous relief. I had been anticipating discharge since speaking with the neurosurgery team on Wednesday. I was ready to leave after spending the night with my poor neighbor.

The neurosurgery team rounds at 5 AM as usual. I was actually awake this time. I essentially told them that I would be leaving today. The young, slight resident politely laughed at one of my bad jokes and agreed that I would be discharged. My blood work looked good, and I would follow up with Dr. Moliterno and Dr. Baehring in the following weeks. The hypertonic saline was stopped. I had one requirement prior to discharge: I had to work with the physical therapy staff to ensure I did not need any additional services when I went home. I asked curtly to have them brought in as soon as possible so I could, "Get the fuck out of here."

A few hours later, a kind young woman came to my door and introduced herself. I said, "Good! You're the one that's going to get me out of here." She laughed and started with some small exercises of simply moving my hands and feet. I stopped after the first two movements and said, "Let's go and do some stairs so we don't waste your time and mine." I stood up and walked past her into the hallway, much to her dismay, but she graciously followed me. As she caught up to me, we chatted and I found that I had graduated high school with her sister. What a small world. We reached the stairs and I bounded up to the first landing, about eight stairs. Then

I turned and walked back down within 30 seconds. I tried to keep any sign of my pounding headache hidden from her, and apparently it worked. She smiled and quickly said, "Oh, you're right. It was a waste of my time. You're all set to go home from my perspective." I told her to write her note quickly so I could, "Get the fuck out of here." She laughed and assured me she would.

I called my wife and packed my things. I looked sadly at my neighbor, who was sleeping in more of a daze than true restful sleep. I thought of all the folks whose rooms I had walked by and thought of their imminent demise. I shook off the thought and faced the opposite direction.

I had been prescribed two medications: Keppra (1000 milligrams twice a day) and a steroid called Decadron (dexamethasone) to keep my brain from swelling. I was soon packed up and had my discharge papers in hand. I thanked the staff and my wife drove me home.

I arrived home and took a shower, the first one since the surgery. It was not as nice as I had expected, given the giant turban-like bandage that encircled my head. Dr. Moliterno directed me to keep the bandage on for five days after surgery. I lamented the bandage, and its canvas was sweltering in the hot June sun.

At the time, my uncle David and his wife, Lauri, were in Connecticut helping my grandmother paint her house. David and Lauri live outside Dallas, Texas, and own a large veterinary clinic. They had planned to come and see my brother and his family and to see my son Vinny's baptism. We had a large Italian feast that night, and I was feeling well other than the nagging headache. I had a glass of wine and ate lots of Nonni's fine Italian home cooking. We all celebrated my discharge from the hospital. It meant so much to have all my family together in one place, laughing and sharing a meal.

Friday, June 28-Sunday, June 30, 2019

The next few days were mostly quiet, or as quiet as life in a large Italian family can be. At our wedding, my wife and I had 320 guests attend—200 of my family members, and 12 of my wife's. The rest were friends from all different facets of our lives: high school, choirs, colleges, camp, Boy Scouts, et cetera.

We had set the day of Sunday, June 30th, 2019 for my second son, Vincent, to be baptized. Family members were coming from near and far to attend the service. My father-in-law, Chip, is an Episcopal priest and so arranged for a stand-in for his congregation on Martha's Vineyard. My brother-in-law, James, who was living in Florida, served as Vinny's godfather. My sister-in-law, MB, served as his godmother. MB, my brother Chris, and their two children, Norah and Sonny, came up from Virginia. We had about 30 other family and friends planning to come to Vinny's baptism. We had set this date months ago, and at the last minute decided that the show must go on, despite brain surgery. Five days after major brain surgery, I removed my turban-bandage, put on a suit, and in the searing heat of summer, sang hymns, baptized my second son, and attended a reception at our church. All with a pounding headache and unable to read quickly enough to follow the lectionary. Fortunately, I knew the words by heart, as I've been a church-goer all my life.

It was a day of relief and merriment. At this point, I was able to show off my new surgical scar, which featured 38 staples in a rectangular shape. I looked like a James Bond villain with my bald head, beard, and huge surgical scar. I was filled with elation that I was still alive and able to speak with all my family, friends, church friends, and well-wishers.

I thanked God in those moments. I felt immense gratitude. I was grateful they had found the tumor and removed it. I was grateful that I'd had a seizure while in bed and not while driving, especially not with my children in the car. I was grateful that it was me with the medical issues, as I knew the system better than anyone else in my family. I was grateful that I'd made it home for such a joyous occasion. My gratitude was overwhelming.

We went home and napped while the kids napped. Later that evening, Caitlin, my sons, and I joined our extended family at Nonni's table, continuing to celebrate the baptism and my triumph after surgery.

Monday, July 1-Sunday, July 2, 2019

The next week began a letdown of all that had transpired over the last couple weeks. The surgery left me with a constant headache, the inability to drive for three months, and an impromptu vacation from work. I was slated to meet with Dr. Baehring on Monday, July 8th. In the meantime, I had some time to relax and try to avoid thinking about the pathology report. I was fairly confident that I would not need further treatment. The initial imaging reports called the mass a "low grade glioma." This essentially means the professionals were surmising the mass was benign and no further intervention would be necessary. I felt confident I would be back to work in another week, as long as my reading improved. The prospect of needing chemotherapy, radiation, and further prolonged chemotherapy was completely off my radar.

My wife and I tried to get back to normalcy. Our son Ralphie was two-and-a-half years old, and Vinny was seven months. They were the same happy-go-lucky kids. However, as is true of children that age, they were prone to temper tantrums, dirty diapers, screaming, crying, and all the craziness you might find in an out-of-control frat party. When you have constant headaches, the normal activities of young children become unrelenting and unavoidably loud.

One evening, Caitlin and I went to a beach in West Haven, Connecticut. In 2004, when we first started dating, we would frequent the restaurant Jimmies of Savin Rock, a quaint seafood joint right on the shore of Long Island Sound. We didn't eat during this visit, but went for memory's sake. There is a long boardwalk that follows the shore with scattered rock cliffs and jetties. People-watching on the boardwalk was a shared pastime, and many walking by us this time looked curious about the giant, angry surgical site and long line of staples in my head. We found a quiet place to sit on the rocks and jetties and speak about memories made years earlier, how much had changed, and what the future may hold, all against the backdrop of a beautiful summer sunset.

The days slowly drifted by as we had a small Fourth of July gathering with some family. We were awaiting some appointments with the oncologist the following week. We were desperately trying to enjoy the days as best we could, however, there was some mild foreboding and anxiety while awaiting a true diagnosis.

On Sunday, an old high school friend invited us to her childhood home for a reunion of sorts. We took the boys so they could have some fun swimming in the pool. Some of the other guests we knew really well, and others we had not seen since high school, 15 years earlier. The folks we knew well and had kept in touch with were mostly sad to hear that Angus had died, but were quickly mesmerized by the story of my awake brain surgery, and thrilled that I was still doing ok. We spoke in quiet whispers and tried not to alert the other folks with whom we hadn't kept in touch. We mostly stayed as optimistic as we could, as we were still awaiting any true information about my diagnosis and prognosis. We were killing time until that Monday appointment, a countdown ticking in our heads all day.

Monday, July 8, 2019

Finally the day came to meet with Dr. Baehring, receive the final diagnosis, and see what was next. At this point, I was cautiously optimistic and thought that all the tests on the tumor would show it to be benign and I would get back to my normal life a few weeks later. The appointment was late in the afternoon, around 4 PM. My wife and I left the kids with my mother and grandmother. As we drove down to New Haven, I incessantly tapped my fingers on my knees, nervous about the news we were to receive.

We arrived at the clinic about an hour prior to my appointment. The clinic is on the eighth floor of the formidable Smilow Cancer Hospital. It is a multispecialty clinic featuring about 30 doctors of various specialties, with their business cards neatly arranged on the wall of the waiting room. I went up to one of the receptionists and gave my name, birthdate, address, and which doctor I had come to see. With kind indifference, the receptionist put a hospital band on my wrist and asked me to sit on one of the cold plastic chairs scattered about the large waiting area. In the corner where we sat, there was a large fish tank with dozens of exotic fish, eels, and other marine life. In a dark twist, there was a dead clown fish lying toward the bottom of the tank, floating idyllically with a small coating of sand on its corpse.

I was called into the back room where vital signs are measured. I got on a scale and realized I had put on some pounds since college, now weighing in at a robust 205 pounds on my 5'8" frame. I had no fever, my pulse rate and oximetry were normal, but my blood pressure was very high: 170/100. The medical assistant asked if I had any symptoms, like headache, double vision, dizziness, or lightheadedness. I responded, "No. I'm about to find out if I have cancer and I'm a little nervous." The MA took my blood pressure again, and it was 166/96. She asked if this was my usual blood pressure. I slowly and pointedly answered, "I'm about to find out if I have cancer and I am very nervous," while looking directly into her eyes. She dropped the subject.

I was brought to a room with more folks waiting to see their respective doctors. The Solarium is a bright room with windows overlooking the healing garden and greater New Haven. I felt like I was in a busy airport, where you get pushed to another stage of your journey, but you are still many hours away from boarding your flight. The room was sparsely decorated, with a small TV in the right upper corner. The audio was out of sync with the news report. There was a shelf with only two items, both hastily placed without much thought: a box of Trivial Pursuit and a box with "The World's Most Difficult Jigsaw Puzzle." I marveled at the brazen choice of these items. One being so trivial and the other an insult to anyone with a brain disability, such as difficulty reading after major brain surgery. Coupled with the TV out of sync, the irony was too thick.

Next, we were brought to an exam room. We waited for another 45 minutes, playing card games to pass the time. Finally, the door opened and in stepped a short Indian man who introduced himself as Dr. Suchin Khanna. He was a resident working with Dr.

Baehring, and given it was early July, it was his second week of practicing oncology. He barely looked into our eyes as he began to speak about chemotherapy and radiation schedules. I interrupted him and told him to slow down, as we didn't even have any diagnosis of cancer nor any results of the tumor pathology taken during the surgery. Dr. Khanna stumbled over his words and apologized as if he had been caught stealing candy from a forbidden jar. It slowly dawned on him that we had no idea of the diagnosis, and he had gone and jumped into explaining treatment. He backtracked and explained, rather poorly, that I had an astrocytoma. He muttered that it was mutated and that this was slightly more favorable. I again interrupted him and asked for a copy of my biopsy report and histological findings. I looked him in his round, brown eyes—which took a second to connect to mine—and slowly, deliberately told him, "Go now and get me the biopsy and pathology reports. I want to see Dr. Baehring. And I am putting you on my haunt list."

"What is a haunt list?" he stammered.

"When I die, you are going to be the first person I haunt. Go get me my reports and the real doctor."

With a nervous laugh, he left the room.

As he left, Caitlin and I looked at each other and started weeping bitterly. The cries of anguish filled the small sterile exam room. We curled up on our respective chairs and held each other. Caitlin, sobbing, said, "This is not what was supposed to happen."

"It will be ok," I choked out, while not believing what I was saying.

I started to compose myself and think clinically. I began to turn off my emotions and look at what the next steps would be. As I had given many cancer diagnoses, I tried to use my clinical judgment and think with a cold, calm, logical approach. I used my education and medical knowledge as a defense mechanism to distance myself from my diagnosis, rather than accept it as a patient.

Since the surgery, I had been reading as much about gliomas as possible. Given my medical knowledge and training, I had a general idea of all the scenarios I could expect to hear when meeting with the oncologist. After getting the diagnosis from Dr. Khanna, I opened UpToDate, an app that gives evidence-based clinical information for providers. I found that with my diagnosis of an anaplastic astrocytoma WHO grade 3 with mutated IDH, I had a life expectancy of eight to ten years. As my tears fell onto my phone, I quickly put it away so Caitlin would not see. She was still holding onto me with shock and horror.

The door opened again after a seemingly eternal 20 minutes. Both Dr. Baehring and Dr. Khanna entered. Dr. Baehring has a commanding presence; he's tall with grey eyes, looking like a five-star general alongside Dr. Khanna, a mere boy scout at his side. Dr. Baehring sat and spoke slowly, his English affected by a German accent. Dr. Khanna handed me my biopsy reports. He laid out my chemotherapy schedule: 42 days of 150 milligrams Temozolomide (Temodar) oral chemotherapy while undergoing radiation, followed by a month off. Then six rounds of five days of Temozolomide with an increased dose, followed by 23 days off. This all comprised a 28-day cycle for my oral chemotherapy. I would essentially be on chemo from August 2019 until April 2020. I had an appointment with Dr. Contessa, a radiation oncologist, in a few days. Dr. Contessa would give me the details of radiation therapy.

Most cancer survivors will tell you that after hearing the "C-word," they don't hear or remember much of the meeting. Clinicians are taught to be mindful of this and try to give as much information as possible to patients before uttering the word "cancer." I found the opposite was true. I remember my discussions with Dr. Baehring and Dr. Khanna with striking detail. I think because I had time to absorb the shock of the diagnosis and then 20 minutes to cry, recompose myself, and recall my medical training and research, I was prepared to hear from Dr. Baehring. I had donned my "medical provider/APRN" hat and was ready to hear about our plan for a mutual patient, instead of thinking of myself as the patient, and hearing the doctors' plan for me.

Dr. Baehring and I spoke frankly and honestly. I was informed again about my diagnosis, anaplastic astrocytoma WHO grade 3 with IDH mutation. I understood the chemotherapy regimen. I would learn more about the radiation schedule from Dr. Contessa, whom I would meet on Thursday. But then I asked the question that most people want to know, and the hardest for doctors to pinpoint, "How much time do I have left, doctor?"

I spoke methodically and asked, "According to my research, I see that the average life expectancy is eight to ten years in these cases. Is that true?"

Dr. Baehring looked me in the eye and said, "Yes, that is true." He went on to cite many factors that would likely add to a longer life expectancy for me: 96% of the tumor removed with surgery, my young age, my overall good health, and the chemo and radiation being especially effective against the IDH mutation.

I missed the last part. All I heard was, "Yes, that is true," but not the silver lining. I heard, "You'll be dead in eight to ten years," which was not exactly the truth. But the mind has a funny way of hearing only certain snippets of information.

Anger is the classic first stage of grief, and it hit like a freight train. I was pissed. *FUCK. I'm going to be dead in ten fucking years!? Fuck you very much, Doc. I have no further questions!*

After the doctors left, I wanted to break everything in that exam room. Tip over the tables, rip off the cupboards, smash the computer, throw the chairs. I especially wanted to take the otoscope off the wall and ring it around Dr. Khanna's scrawny neck for giving me the bad news in such a poor way. Anger swelled. I'm sure my blood pressure was even higher than it had been at sign-in.

A kind nurse came in shortly after to have me sign papers to receive my Temozolomide prescription. It was a double-sided form explaining the risks and benefits of the medications. It was simply a standard consent form, not too different from any medical procedure. I signed the form on autopilot. Obviously, I was going to take the chemo and follow the oncologist's directions. I had plenty of resources for medical providers that I could read later. I didn't have any other questions. I wanted out. Caitlin and I gravely walked out of the exam room and to the elevators.

We drove home in silence. No music played, no voices spoke; there were only dim, sorrowful breaths. I did not have my fingers tapping on my knees any longer. I was in a quiet rage. Thoughts were cascading through my head. *What will I do in the next ten-ish years before I die? What will happen to my kids and wife when I'm gone? Will I ever get back to work?* I had never been so disoriented and so anxious about what I would do next. My medical training and knowledge of the complications that cancer patients suffer. Thoughts of immunocompromised patients reduced to walking corpses before finally dying in their hospice rooms. My thoughts bounced to God. *Was this a test? Was it my destiny? Was it punishment?*

Then thoughts of what I had imagined my life's plan ought to be. *I was supposed to die of heart disease in my 80s, like everyone else in my family—not brain cancer while in my 30s!*

My mind was still spinning when we arrived home. Caitlin went to help my mother get the kids ready for bath and bed. I did not want to even look at my children, because they were not only screaming with elation in the bath, but I couldn't bear the thought of never seeing them again.

I quietly and quickly told my mother and grandmother that the tumor was malignant and my grim prognosis. I went out on my deck to spend some time alone.

My father arrived shortly after I sat down on the deck. I told him the news, and his eyes welled with tears as he uttered, "Oh, fuck." We embraced, shedding small tears. He briefly spoke about life and death and what the future may hold. He went inside to help the children get ready for bed. The children went to bed, and my father, mother, and grandmother sat with disbelief as I recounted the events at the neuro-oncology appointment. We held each other, and Caitlin and I asked to be alone. They left with tears in their eyes.

I grabbed a bottle of Jameson whiskey, poured a generous glass, and reached for an old pack of stale cigarettes. I had smoked intermittently in college and would indulge two or three times a year if out for a long night of drinking. I saved a pack that I had bought two years earlier for a camping trip with some friends. I sat in an Adirondack chair and looked over the side of my deck, which overlooks a 40-acre nature preserve. Several tall dead ash trees towered over the woods. A few years earlier, there was a blight which had killed off most of the ash trees, which were just waiting to fall down and gradually return to the soil. I sipped whiskey and let my mind continue to wander about my circumstances. I thought of the dead ash trees and my own imminent demise.

After sitting for about an hour, I called my brother, who insisted on returning to Connecticut the following week to be with us. Since being in the hospital during most of their visit two weeks earlier, we agreed that we should have a true vacation. They planned to spend the next week in Connecticut and we would find fun things to do with the kids. As the sun went down, I continued my sorrowful evening with more whiskey and mindless TV. I was overcome by despair and was crossing over to the denial stage of grief. I threw away the rest of the stale pack of cigarettes and cried myself to sleep.

Tuesday, July 9-Wednesday, July 10, 2019

Over the next two days, I functioned in a dream like state. I made blurry-eyed phone calls to several entities. First, I started making arrangements with my boss, Dr. Mohammed Shams. I explained the diagnosis and the anticipated chemo and radiation schedules. I would be transitioned to a leave of absence and start short-term disability, which would continue until the end of December that year. His kindness and help through all the process was exceptional; he was understanding and supportive, determined that I take the time I needed to heal and eventually rejoin the team at Midstate.

I had to make calls to cancel other plans. Since I had already maxed out my insurance deductible, I was under the assumption that the costs of my medical care would be covered. However, as I was employed by Hartford Healthcare, my Aetna health insurance plan considered YNHH an out-of-network provider. I made several calls to Aetna and spoke with their "healthcare advocates." I dryly told them that they would be getting more huge bills from YNHH. They assured me that my medical coverage would continue and my care would be covered. An estimation of the costs associated with my care—ambulance transport, ER work up, laboratory tests, imaging tests, consultations with three different services, hospital stay, major brain surgery, and ICU care—at this point would be approximately $550,000.

In my anger, I started to lash out at other people I spoke to over the phone. I had a vasectomy scheduled for August; obviously, I wasn't about to undergo any procedure after brain surgery and impending chemo and radiation. I called the clinic and spoke to an unsuspecting receptionist in order to cancel my appointment. I told her, "I am dying of brain cancer, so I don't want to cut off my balls." She stated with a soft and genuine voice, "I'm so sorry to hear that...." I rudely interrupted with a pointed, "Save your platitudes. We all die at some point." I hung up the phone immediately after confirming the canceled appointments.

I also called my student loan lender. After graduating from Yale School of Nursing, I had about $190,000 in student loan debt. I had been paying back the loans with sums much larger than the minimum payment. I spoke to another kind receptionist and said, "Before you have to rip this money from my cold, dead hands, or my wife's as she sobs, I want to switch my loans into fucking forbearance." She gracefully accepted my request, and I had my payments reduced to the minimum.

I stayed in the anger stage of grief for a while. I was pointedly rude to people on the phone, often using the aforementioned phrases. I screamed at robocalls, both automated and human, with profanity and curses that would make Satan himself blush. I was reckless, drinking lots of alcohol. I was smoking a truly heroic amount of cannabis, easily obtained in Massachusetts, where it can be legally purchased for recreational use. My excuse was, "I have fucking brain cancer and I'm not working. I can do whatever I want!"

Fortunately, my wife was both compassionate and stern. She would allow me to drive short distances, which was illegal in Connecticut until three months of being seizure-free. I never drove with the children in the car, nor while drinking or smoking. She was gracious to see that I was grief-stricken, and coping with booze and drugs was an adequate short-term response.

Every day was a fog of increasing headaches and stress. Just touching my head near the surgical scar caused a thunder clap throughout my head. Loud high-pitched noises would hit like an ice pick into my temple. The continued pain coupled with two young boys created an epic slog through every day, and it was only getting worse.

Thursday, July 11, 2019

Caitlin and I returned to YNHH to meet with the radiation oncologist. Their office in YNHH is on the lower level of the Smilow Cancer Center, in the basement. The waiting area is in stark contrast to the eighth floor multispecialty center, with the exception of a fish tank. The lower level's fish tank was enormous, with an even larger assortment of fish and aquatic life, centered in the middle of the room, and visible on all sides. There were no dead fish, thankfully. There was a small kitchenette with assorted coffee, tea, and crackers with peanut butter. Tucked in the corner was an alcove with two computers and some large puzzles awaiting completion. For such a grim activity of radiation, this was a surprisingly warm spot.

I checked in, admired the large room, and surveyed the 30 or so patients and visitors who were seated around the room. Caitlin and I were called to a room by a friendly MA who took my weight and other vital signs. We were given a welcome packet with loads of information and pictures of happy faces in sunny places, a sickening display for someone recently diagnosed with cancer and awaiting the sentence of radiation. The MA left and we perused the welcome packet.

A few minutes later, a kind, short, blonde woman who looked like she was about 20 years old walked in and introduced herself as a resident of Dr. Contessa. She said she had some questions before outlining the next steps and procedure. Remembering my horrific interaction with Dr. Khanna, I was very short with this second resident. I knew what she was going to ask, and rattled off exactly what she would write in her note. After I had finished, I asked her, "What do you want to be when you grow up?" I normally ask this question in a light, yet condescending tone to students who see me during their training. She smiled and coolly answered, "Radiation oncologist."

She then started to explain the process of radiation. Essentially, I would have another MRI one month after surgery, followed by a CT scan to pinpoint exactly where the radiation would be targeting. This would ensure the maximum amount of radiation would be directed at the correct spot and destroy the remaining cancer cells, those which were not removed during surgery. The resident finished explaining the procedures and asked if we had any questions. "No questions, thank you." She left the exam room and stated that Dr. Contessa would be in shortly.

Dr. Contessa entered the room a few minutes later. He sat and introduced himself and said, "I just spoke with the resident and would like to follow up on a few items. What did you gather from what she said?" This was the first time an attending physician had asked what we'd understood from the interaction with the resident. I started my usual speech about my role in medicine as a hospitalist, and quickly gave a recap of what I would be enduring over the next few months. About halfway through my diatribe and intermittent word-finding difficulties, he held up his hand and gently interrupted, "I see you know quite a bit about this, but for the sake of your wife,

and so I don't miss anything, I would like to clarify a few things."
He again slowly outlined the MRI and CT scan plan, how the
radiation would be dosed and calculated, and what side effects could
be expected. After he finished, he turned his whole body to face
Caitlin and kindly asked her if she had any questions. She asked
what signs and symptoms would point to serious danger. He
explained that I may need a course of steroids if there were large
amounts of swelling in the brain. We had no other questions and
returned to the waiting area to schedule the MRI and CT
appointments.

I liked Dr. Contessa right from the start. His cool, calm, and
confident demeanor was a welcome change to what had transpired
three days prior at Dr. Baehring's office. His resident was competent
and knew how to speak with patients. The way he both respected my
medical knowledge, yet spoke with authority and expertise, was
truly a blessing that I needed at the time. The way he spoke to Caitlin
was empathetic, especially the way he spoke to her before asking if
I had questions. This encounter was a breath of fresh air during a
dismal time.

Wednesday, July 17, 2019

About three weeks after surgery, I had my follow up with Dr. Moliterno. We wanted to bring some sort of gift for all she had done for us. What does one give to someone who stuck big sharp knives into your brain and kept you from dying? Given our mutual Italian ancestry, we settled on some Italian pastries from Lucibello's Pastry Shop in New Haven, about a mile from the hospital. I also insisted on writing her a thank you note; this took me a fairly long time to draft, edit, and rewrite.

We arrived early to the same multispecialty floor where we'd seen Dr. Baehring at Smilow Cancer Hospital. The dead clown fish had been removed from the fish tank. I tried not to think about how unceremonial its disposal must have been.

I was called and brought in for vital sign measurements and general screening questions. We were then escorted to the Solarium. I again scoffed at "The World's Most Difficult Jigsaw Puzzle." As I was thinking of creative ways to destroy the puzzle and other items in the room, my name was called, and we were brought to one of the exam rooms.

Immediately after entering the room, Dr. Moliterno joined us. She hugged both of us and sat on the rolling stool. She graciously accepted the pastries. Her demeanor changed, and a sorrowful expression crossed her face. She asked if we had heard about the biopsy reports. "Yes, we heard," I quickly replied, not wanting to relive the horror of the initial reception of the report. She said she was sorry and wished she had better news. She reiterated her optimism, as she was excited and proud to have been able to remove so much of the tumor.

She had an RN with her to help remove the 38 staples. They had healed well and I had no complications nor pain, other than following an occasional bump on the car door or a grab by one of my kids. She removed all the staples but caused almost no pain. I asked if I could now shave my head, returning to the bald head I'd sported since 2014. She gave me a stern "No." She told me she'd spoken with Dr. Baehring and was so happy that he was my neuro-oncologist. She and many others had been raving about him and his competency and expertise in treating people with brain tumors. After my outpatient meeting, I was not so sure.

She asked if we had any questions, and then complemented Caitlin, saying this was the first time they had spoken without Caitlin shedding any tears. I asked about my difficulty reading. She sighed and told me, "When I was training at Memorial Sloan-Kettering in New York City, we would say 'if there is no disability after removal of the tumor, then we did not take enough tumor out.'" She continued by saying my reading might improve after the trauma and swelling from surgery receded. The timeline for healing could not be given, as it depended on a number of factors, such as overall health, other comorbidities, concurrent chemo or radiation, etc. When would I be able to read again? Maybe six weeks, maybe six months, maybe six years? Maybe never?

As long as I had no other brain tumors or anything that would necessitate neurosurgery, I would not need her services any longer. We again thanked her profusely and sarcastically said, "I hope we never have to meet again."

However, I was also taken aback by not being able to shave my head, and my anger surged. I wanted to get back to some semblance of my normal life. My shaved bald head was a big part of that normal life. Now I had a bald top with hair growing on the sides and back of my head. I had been looking forward to regaining some control, which had been stripped away after the first seizure. Returning to my hairstyle of choice was the bargaining stage of grief.

I was also perturbed at her lackadaisical answer to my reading troubles. I was barely able to read my sons' children's books! How was I supposed to read medical charts and interpret all the data that would enable me to do my job? I couldn't go back to work if I couldn't fucking read! And nothing but a lame story about not cutting enough? This is bullshit. Anger and depression seethed during this grief stage. Then these feelings mixed with bargaining as I remembered that it was still nothing short of a miracle that I was able to even read a little, let alone was alive, talking, able to comprehend speech, and had no physical deficits, other than constant headaches. Guilt followed anger. I felt guilt for being so enraged at Dr. Moliterno, who literally saved my life with amazing skill and expertise. How could I feel any resentment? Feelings like this would continue throughout my journey.

I cannot overstate how grateful I am to Dr. Moliterno for her work on my brain. Although I was angry about losing my ability to read, I was glad I had no other deficits. I was grateful for the successful surgery and the skill of her work. It is hard to put into words how much you appreciate someone who literally swooped in and saved your life.

Thursday, July 25, 2019

I drove myself to all the appointments I had on Thursday. We didn't have any childcare options that day, so Caitlin stayed home with the kids. I drove recklessly to a YNHH satellite facility in North Haven, where I received an MRI of the brain with and without contrast. This MRI was exactly one month after surgery and would give a precise view of how my brain was healing. The contrast would elucidate any residual tumor/cancer findings. The test was fairly quick, and then I went to New Haven to have a CT scan and meet with Dr. Contessa.

The CT scan was completed at the lower level in the radiation suite. I was brought into the CT scanner. I lay supine on the hard surface of the scanner table, which was moved into the doughnut-shaped scanner. Afterward, the radiation technologists came into the room. I was to be fitted for a mask that would encircle my face. In the CT scan, the technologists used a plastic substance called Aquaplast. It was warmed in hot water and then applied to my face, ears, and the back of my head. Over 30 minutes, the warm plastic solidified and hardened to make a plastic cast of my face. Various small holes dotted the mask. Imagine a wiffle ball with smaller holes stretched and pressed tightly onto your face. The mask was so tight on my face that I was happy I didn't suffer from claustrophobia. Using the images from the CT and MRI, the hardened mask is marked to show precisely how to line up the radiation delivery. A computer is used to calculate exactly how and where the radiation will be delivered to have the maximum effect, all while preserving sensitive areas, such as eyes, ears, and neck. My calculations dictated a schedule of 33 sessions of radiation therapy to be completed Monday through Friday at 9 AM. This schedule would start a few weeks later, on August 12th, and last for seven weeks.

The initial setup for the mask took about 45 minutes. I then scheduled a dry run the week prior to the first session. This dry run was a successful endeavor of fitting the plastic mask back on my face, lining up the guide lasers, and angling the movable table so the radiation machine would deliver the radiation exactly where the computer had calculated.

Starting on August 12th, I would meet with Dr. Contessa weekly. I was anxious to start so that I could finish sooner. However, the general guidelines for initiation of chemo and radiation recommend beginning these treatments about six weeks after surgery. The rationale for this timeline being that it would allow for the body to heal after the trauma of the surgery prior to the bombardment of the chemo and radiation. I had to wait a few more weeks.

Waiting for August 12th

The waiting was brutal. I would cross through every stage of grief each day. I would be in denial that I even had cancer, as I felt ok, but also felt frustrated that I wasn't getting any real treatment yet. Looking down the barrel at months of burning radiation into my head and chemical pills. I was angry almost all the time. Little things would throw me into a rage. I would ask God, "Why me?" and literally bargain for my life. I was not my usual happy, even-keeled self, but rather stuck in a deep depression. Yet I was constantly accepting my fate; as every living person must die, so will I. And then the cycle would repeat. This was only a foretaste of what was to come, as I hadn't even started the impending harsh treatment of chemo and radiation.

The waves of emotion were crushing. I would have mood swings and crash through different emotions. As a staid clinician and provider of medical care, I was at both an advantage and disadvantage. Memories would surface of all the people I had seen perish from cancer. I thought of the literally hundreds of death certificates I had signed. I thought of the suffering I'd witnessed and wondered how I could now be on that side of death and disease. And at only 32 years old! Was this a punishment for something I had done or not done? Had I stopped CPR too early on someone who may have otherwise lived? Had I not been fast enough giving some drug or treatment, which then led to someone's demise? I went through thousands of scenarios of people I had treated and conjured the ones lost. I asked for forgiveness vaguely, as I didn't really know if I was at fault.

I would think of my wife and kids and how they would be without me. At least I had life insurance. But would I ever live to play catch with my sons, teach them how to drive, watch them graduate high school or college? Would I see them get married and have children of their own?

I thought of the songs I wanted at my funeral and how my obituary would be written. Although I never wrote anything down, I had a very good idea of what my funeral would be like. I stopped myself from writing my final funeral wishes on multiple occasions. This was partially because I was still having trouble reading and writing, but also because I thought if I did, I would lose hope and lose the battle.

The angry phone calls continued. I would often tell the recipient my "dying of brain cancer" situation, followed by me snarling, "Save your platitudes," before they could give some sort of apology. The anger inside me loved the line, "Save your platitudes." It is a perfect way to invalidate any kind gesture that some unsuspecting well-wisher might give. An incredibly rude tactic, yet at the time it was a powerful rebuke to anyone with whom I was frustrated.

I continued to fuel my rage with alcohol and cannabis use. Obviously, this was the worst possible coping mechanism I could have employed. While running and driving had been some of my favorites, now I could not go for a run, and I couldn't drive. I was stuck home with two screaming kids. I wasn't working, was just killing time until treatment, and so I found drinking and smoking helped. Or at least I thought so at the time.

There were some breaks in the storm clouds. Bristol Hospital staff had written personal notes to encourage me and collected a large sum of money to help with my expenses. Midstate Medical Center staff also sent words of encouragement and donated large sums to help us. A huge outpouring of support enveloped me and my family, which brightened some of the darkest days.

My wife and I had the opportunity to escape for a day to go to Boston to watch a Red Sox game. The Sox lost 9-4 against the Tampa Bay Rays. It was a somber date in the city, appropriate for my mood. We had offers to attend BBQs, house warmings, and other get-togethers during that August. We went to one such housewarming and realized quickly we had nothing good to report about our summer plans. "Hi! It's so good to see you! How has your summer been?!" our friends asked. "Oh, fucking miserable. The dog died and I have brain cancer. Thanks for asking! Fuck you very much!" We weren't exactly the life of the party.

We did get a new dog during this time—a lovable, 75-pound pit bull rescue named Whit. Instead of googling images of brain tumors, Caitlin and I perused dog rescue sites. Most other dog lovers encouraged us to take the plunge and get a new dog soon after the death of Angus, as it would only bring more life, vitality, and love into our home. Our whole family met Whit before she came to live with us, and she was such a lovely addition to our home. Miraculously very tolerant of the young kids, having had a litter of her own in the past. She became an instant part of the family, especially devoted to me. She basically never left my side since she arrived. Dogs know when you are sick, and Whit was no exception. She knew I needed rescue as much as she did.

After treating so many patients with a variety of illnesses and trauma, you cannot help but view your own medical issues in a clinical way. As I mentioned, medical training essentially directs you to find the first thing that will kill the patient. This is in order to rule it out or fix it, then triage the next thing that will kill the patient and fix it or rule it out. Deeply ingrained in me, this particular thought process of assuming the worst-case scenario started to infect how I thought of my own health. This is colloquially known as medical student syndrome, where medical students perceive themselves to be experiencing the symptoms of a disease which they are studying. Although a rational person and a board-certified medical professional, I couldn't help but start thinking of other plagues that were lurking under my skin.

My bout of medical student syndrome peaked the week before I was going to start chemo and radiation. I had noticed that there was a small piece of suture protruding from the side of my surgical incision. When Dr. Moliterno finished removing the tumor, the team had to sew up my head. They used a number of dissolvable sutures to close up the incision, followed by the 38 staples that fully closed the outer layer of scalp. One of the sutures was poking out of my skin all of a sudden. I tried to pick at it, but it hurt and sent shock waves through my head as I pulled. I started to panic and have completely irrational thoughts.

Didn't they use dissolvable sutures in my head? It was mostly staples in there, so how could this be a suture? Oh God, this is the start of a huge abscess! My brain could be infected. I could be going septic! IF I PULL THIS OUT, WILL I UNRAVEL MY HEAD AND BRAIN LIKE A FUCKING SWEATER?!

I called Dr. Moliterno's office and got an appointment with one of her colleagues the next day. I panicked all night. Wondering if my radiation and chemo would be delayed or if I'd have to go back to the OR, as the nurse who scheduled the appointment had suggested.

Fear and anxiety are powerful things, especially after seeing the worst medical conditions routinely. The doubt and apprehension can be crippling. It robs you of your rational, educated, and scientific thought process and puts your mind in a place where you cannot simply examine your situation and then make the next best decision. It was especially oppressive now that I did not feel strong and healthy. Rather I felt like a weak and debilitated cancer patient on the brink of death. All my rational thought was ripped away by fear and anxiety.

I arrived at the eighth floor multispecialty center the next day. I was brought back to the same exam room #4, where I had been given my diagnosis. I shuddered in the cold, sterile exam room. A few minutes later, an older neurosurgeon colleague of Dr. Moliterno entered the room. I told him, "I think there is a suture hanging out of my head, but I can't really see it." I made sure to leave out the irrational idea of my head unraveling like a sweater. He looked at the area, grabbed a pair of tweezers, and effortlessly pulled out a small 1 cm dissolving suture, saying, "Yeah, this happens sometimes. No problem!"

No further anxiety, at least for now. I looked at him sheepishly and said, "Thanks for allowing me to waste your time today." He laughed and hardily slapped my shoulder, saying, "Haha! I like you! Thanks! Be safe."

Later that night, I vowed not to be taken by fear and anxiety any longer. I needed to be stronger and get ready for the marathon ahead. I needed to prove to myself that I could overcome some pain with brazen action. I had a small skin tag on my face, on the right side of my nose. I took a pair of surgical scissors and snipped the skin tag right off. I wiped it down with alcohol and put gauze and ice on the wound to staunch the bleeding. I figured if I could undergo brain surgery and that silly appointment for suture removal, I owed it to myself to take off that measly skin tag.

I could manage the brain surgery, pounding headaches, screaming kids, and a cocktail of anger, fear, anxiety, grief, and irrationality. I was ready to jump into the trenches of chemo and radiation.

Monday, August 12, 2019

The day had arrived. Chemo and radiation would start today. My regimen of Temozolomide was 155 milligrams daily for 42 days (six weeks). This oral form of chemotherapy is the standard of care for brain cancer, as it penetrates the blood-brain barrier better than IV agents. In addition, it is easier to administer as a pill rather than have an IV infusion. I would wake up and take an 8 milligram Ondansetron (Zofran) pill, a prophylactic anti-nausea medication. Half an hour later, I would take the 155 milligrams of Temozolomide (Temodar), which came in four pills: one 140 mg tablet, and three 5 mg tablets. Then I had to wait an hour until I could eat or drink in order to mitigate nausea and vomiting. The first few days I felt fine, but I felt worse if I didn't start the regimen early in the morning so that I could get breakfast and coffee earlier rather than later. I would take the Zofran around 6 AM, the Temozolomide at 6:30 AM, and breakfast/coffee at 7:30 AM.

The first radiation session took place on a hot summer morning. My uncle, Kevin, would drive me to my appointment, as my wife and I agreed that the 25 minutes of city driving while undergoing chemo and radiation was not only illegal, but foolhardy and downright stupid. We arrived at the valet parking entrance and were greeted by a man named Ryan, a guy in his mid-twenties with a thick beard and kind demeanor. He was responsible for all the radiation patients' cars. This was the only place in New Haven where one didn't need a parking sticker nor payment. It was all covered by Smilow. I chuckled to myself and thought I must be in bad shape if the City of

New Haven was allowing us to park for free. Ryan would park our car and knew everyone's name and car. He was a warm light in a dark place each morning we saw him for the next seven weeks.

The actual radiation sessions took about 10-15 minutes. I would be escorted in my street clothes to the hard table surface. The Aquaplast mask that had been molded to my face and head would be applied. The table would angle so I would be tilted slightly with my head towards the floor and listing toward the right. Then the radiation machine would be brought close to my face and guide lasers would line up with my mask. The mask was so tight on my face. I had to close my eyes once it was applied and could not open them because my eyelids were pressed down. The staff would exit the room, and I would hear the machine starting up with an increasing whir. The table would twitch and move slightly. Then after a few clicks, the radiation would start. It always followed the same path, one prescribed by the computer. There were three buzzing sounds with movement of the actual radiation machine above me. There was also a blue guide laser that would shine into my eyes, despite them being closed. After the three buzzing sounds and radiation treatment, the heavy lead door would open and the staff would unhook the mask. I was able to sit up and be escorted out. That was the end of one session, only lasting 10-15 minutes. Only 32 left to go.

Depending on which type of cancer or reason for radiation therapy, one could have a variety of side effects associated with the radiation treatment. The most common complaint is fatigue. I was on both chemotherapy and radiation, so I cannot be certain what side effects were caused by radiation alone. I am fairly sure that the headaches, fatigue, and sensitivity to high-pitched sounds were exacerbated by the radiation. In addition, I would get an odd sense of taste and smell that was akin to the acrid smell of burning wire. This taste would stay for about two hours after radiation, but then return randomly throughout the day. It is hard to eat when your mouth tastes like an electrical fire. I also noticed that blue light would trigger headaches and the acrid taste. For example, if I saw a police car on the side of the road, especially at night, I would immediately have a worsening headache and acrid taste that would last for at least two hours.

For the first two weeks of this treatment plan, I felt pretty good. I was certainly eating less, as I would have the sensation of fullness after eating very little food. This is called early satiety. I started to lose some weight. I had certainly been overweight, and could have lost a few pounds, but chemo and radiation proved to be the worst diet plan ever. I was mildly fatigued, but still keeping up with the kids, housework, cooking, and other activities of daily living. I was also keeping a steady diet of beer, whiskey, and cannabis. The world would again crash down around me once I started to think about my future. It was like the dark of night sweeping across the sky to chase away the sun.

Saturday, August 24, 2019

Two weeks in, and I was still feeling pretty good on chemo and radiation. It was the weekend, so I only had to take the chemo pills. No radiation treatments on the weekends. My sister-in-law, Bridget, and her husband, Pablo, were visiting from Florida and staying through the next week. I was feeling fine, and we all went to a nearby park with assorted farm animals to entertain the kids. We came home and hung around outside as I started up the grill to make dinner. I still felt fine, especially considering the amount of cannabis I was on and beer I was drinking while making dinner. I had just sneaked another hit off my cannabis vape pen and was feeling the high creep through me.

I was at the grill and spoke to Caitlin saying, "passavative." I had a little laugh and tried again to say, "I'm going to put the pork chops on the grill," but out of my mouth came, "passavative." Caitlin and I went into the house. She told Bridget, "Watch the kids. I have to figure out what is going on."

In the kitchen, I kept repeating, "It's passavative!" In my head, I knew what I wanted to say, but the words just were not coming out that way.

Caitlin frantically asked, "What happened? Did you just smoke weed? Or do I need to call the ambulance?"

She wrote "yes" and "no" on a nearby legal pad, and asked me to point to my answer. "Are you going to have a seizure?"

I pointed to "yes" and then "no." I panicked. "Passavative, passavative, passavative," I replied. With that, I grabbed a Keppra pill and swallowed it as fast as I could.

It was too late. I felt my body contort and pull to the right. Caitlin caught me and helped me to the couch, where I vomited. The next thing I remember was the police and ambulance personnel standing over me. I looked up and a different friend from my Campion Ambulance days was standing over me. I tried to say, "Hi, Jay," to the paramedic I had worked with years earlier. Instead, "passavative" emerged from my lips. Again, my body contorted and I felt the second seizure. I awoke later in the postictal state, and looked at an IV in my left arm as the blue sky above me rolled by. I realized I was on the stretcher, and was then loaded into the ambulance. I slowly regained some consciousness and looked at Jay. The only word I could say was, "Fuck."

As my mind was racing, I thought of a time many years ago when Jay and I were giving a man CPR while blood poured from the stretcher onto the floor. The young man had been thrown from a motorcycle into a brick wall and suffered severe traumatic injuries. He lost pulses when we picked him up at the scene, and we tried to resuscitate him all the way to the hospital. Alas, he was pronounced dead at the ER. *Was this going to be my fate? Was I going to make it out of this ambulance alive? Did the last person on this stretcher live?*

In my postictal state, I looked at Jay while I lay on the stretcher. I thought of the story and wanted to recount it to Jay, but the only thing I could say was, "Fuck." He looked down at me with concern in his eyes. I gave a thumbs up and put my head down on the stretcher. A few minutes later, he asked again if I was ok. I tried to answer, and again my head and body contorted as I began to seizure for the third time. Jay yelled to the EMT driver and my wife, "He's seizing again." Then quiet darkness.

At the YNHH ER, my wife had to recount my medical history to the doctors. She gave the best information and was able to relay all that the ER staff needed to know. They asked Jay which meds he had given. "Six of Ativan and ten of Versed." The ER staff froze in shock, "Ten of Versed?!" Jay gave a shrug and said, "I knew his history, and I wanted to stop him from seizing." I'm glad he did.

Lorazepam (Ativan) is a benzodiazepine used for anxiety disorders but also to stop seizure activity. Usually, you start by giving 2 milligrams to see if it stops the seizures, and then increase the dosage as necessary. Midazolam (Versed) is a much more powerful benzodiazepine usually used for sedation in the ICU before a breathing tube is put in (intubation), or in the OR as anesthesia prior to a surgical procedure. An off-label use of 10 milligrams IV can be used in refractory seizures, but usually causes the patient to stop breathing, and they often need to be intubated. Fortunately, I was protecting my airway and avoided intubation. I had learned a lot from Jay when working with him, and I was really glad he was the paramedic that picked me up that day.

The next few hours were a complete blur. I was in and out of sleep. A generalized (aka grand mal seizure) saps a large amount of energy, and has been described as running a marathon within a few minutes. After the three seizures and the large amount of sedating medication, I was absolutely exhausted. I would sleep for a few hours, then would wake up and not be able to speak except to say the word, "Fuck." Later that evening, around 11 PM, the ER folks had consulted with the neurology team and made a decision. My speech had not returned, so the ER doctors had decided to admit me to the neurology service.

I remember hearing the conversation the neurology resident had with Caitlin and my father. I heard the word "admit" and I angrily wanted to refuse, but I wasn't able to speak. I started to thrash in the bed and rip off my EKG wires, tear out my IV, and grab the bedside rails to shake them violently. I screamed, "Fuck!" as I had no other words to say. I couldn't convey that I did not want to be admitted nor spend any more time in the hospital. My father and Caitlin had to try to calm me down. I sat on the chair and panted like a caged animal. I was finally too exhausted to fight any more. I slowly moved back to the bed and fell asleep moments after I lay down.

A little later, a nurse came to put me back on the EKG monitor. "Fuck off. My EKG has been fine," I said. As she insisted on putting on the EKG monitor, I realized that I was starting to be able to speak a few more words. The next word I uttered was a sheepish, "Sorry." I then rolled over and allowed her to reapply the EKG tabs.

Later, the same nurse came in to start a new IV. I looked at the pink wrapping of the 20 gauge IV. I grunted and started to say, "No, no, not...FUCK. Not that one." The nurse looked puzzled, and started to assure me that I needed an IV. "I know, but...FUCK...ummmmm." I gestured for a pen, and wrote it on the bed sheet. 18g. A larger bore needle so I could receive interventions faster. This was also my favorite needle to give to anyone who would come to the ER. My rationale at that time was if you need IV meds in the ER, you need a large bore needle in your arm. I figured I should receive the same care I had given to so many people over the years.

Sunday, August 25, 2019

Throughout that Sunday, I was in a stupor, sleeping over 36 hours since the initial seizure. Caitlin and my father sat vigil at my bedside from the time I got to the ER, around 6 PM Saturday, through Sunday evening around 8 PM. They took shifts, as I could not speak for myself. Caitlin called a friend who lived in New Haven and crashed at her apartment for a few hours early Sunday, then returned later that morning. My father went home to sleep for a few hours and then came back later that afternoon. My mother was with Bridget and Pablo watching the kids.

A troop of neurology residents and fellows flowed in and out through the morning. They would speak with either my dad or Caitlin, barely addressing me. I could not speak very much. I could write only a few misspelled words on a hospital note pad. It was more frustrating than anything you could imagine. I had a medical degree from Yale, I could understand everything that the residents and doctors were discussing. I was usually the translator for my family members when they spoke to medical personnel, but now I was essentially bedridden without the ability to speak, read, or write.

While still waiting for a hospital room, I was hooked up to an electroencephalogram (EEG). Thirty electrodes were glued to my head, all connected to wires which led to a large portable computer. The wires detect brain cells communicating with each other and then display the results on a continuous graph. This continuous graph can show if the brain is functioning normally or if there are other signs of abnormalities. When I was initially hooked up, I was having approximately one to five mini seizures every minute, or 60-300 mini seizures every hour.

FUCK. No wonder I can't speak.

I was given more Keppra to try and slow the progression of seizures, but it barely made any difference on the EEG. The mini seizures were not like the initial seizures that had prompted my ambulance transport. Instead, they would give me the inability to speak, read, and write, accompanied by some slight confusion, and then add to my exhaustion.

I was finally moved to the South Pavilion 6-3, on the Epilepsy Unit, around 5 PM. I was still having multiple mini seizures, and the EEG was still attached to my head. I was placed in a private room where the EEG machine would plug into the wall. There was a camera above me which monitored me in the event of a seizure, or if I had a change on my EEG, or if I did not follow proper procedure. Getting out of bed unassisted was not following their procedure. Contrary to my hospital stay before the surgery, I was now on lock down.

My father had just arrived when the neurology team spoke about adding a new medication to help stop my seizures. We were going to try Phenytoin (Dilantin), a fairly common anti-seizure medication that is usually a second-line agent for continued seizure activity. I gave a thumbs up and my dad said, "Ok." I was given the Dilantin.

Minutes later came a sensation like I was being pushed into a sauna with warmth flowing over my whole body. My eyes opened, and I was ripped from my continued dozing. Then the itching started. Itching so fierce it made me want to claw my skin off. Starting on my chest, I just started scratching. Harder and harder I clawed now all over my body.

"Itching! Fuck! Recon...FUCK...read...FUCK...REACTION!" I yelled for my father and tried to convey that I was itching all over, which meant I was likely having a reaction to the Dilantin. The horror of patients I'd seen flashed through my brain. Next step: throat closing, hypotension, respiratory and cardiac arrest. Now panicking, a flurry of nurses came into the room. The Dilantin was stopped.

Fortunately, I calmed down and had no worsening reactions. No throat closings, no wheezing or need for steroids, no intubation. The neurology resident came to check on things. I was given 50 milligrams of Benadryl. Caitlin walked in right after all the commotion. A different drug, Topiramate (Topamax), would be tried instead of Dilantin. We all agreed. It was given to me around 8 PM with no side effects. The nurse who stayed by my side well beyond her shift time asked if I was doing ok. I looked at her and said, "Just check the orbits...fuck...obituaries." She was horrified at the comment, but I did my best to assure her I was joking. Despite all of this, although I could barely express my thoughts, I was keeping an impressive monologue of inappropriate humor in my head.

The Benadryl kicked in, and I started to doze off as Caitlin and my father continued to talk quietly in my room. They would ask me a few questions intermittently, but then were asked to leave as visiting hours ended. They left around 9 PM, and I fell into a deep sleep shortly after.

Monday, August 26, 2019

I was shaken awake around 6 AM to bright lights and a woman who chirped her name so fast I couldn't even hear it. A needle was forced into my arm for labs. She was such a flurry of activity and labs and vitals that I couldn't take it in. I started to get up from the bed, but was startled by the bed alarm—a shrill, loud, and obnoxious ring which not only scared me but sent shock waves through my head. I tried to sit back down, but a veritable platoon of nurses and MAs flooded into my room. "Sit down, sit down!" they all barked. I tried to utter an apology, but only managed to sputter, "Fuck...I'm sitting down. I didn't mean to..." and I held up my hands in surrender.

One MA stayed with me to change the bed sheets and allowed me to walk to the bathroom with her assistance. After about 36 hours of sitting in a bed, I was quite stiff. I could barely walk and was sore all over. At 32 years old, I felt like a 90-year-old, and wondered if I should be using a walker. I was also unsteady, given my head was still attached to the EEG, a large gauze swatch securing it. It is a truly humbling experience to have a woman—who is not your wife—hold your arm as you take a piss.

I hobbled back to the freshly-made bed and lay down. I was exhausted from the ten-foot walk from bed to bathroom and back to bed. The bed alarm was armed. The MA left, and I closed my eyes and sighed. I looked around the room and up at the camera. I felt like I was a trained prison guard who had just been locked up himself. I was on the wrong side of the bars now.

Glance at the clock on the wall: 6:30 AM. Breakfast orders start at 7:00 at YNHH. I grabbed the remote and turned on the TV. It opened to a local news station. A chipper news anchor started with a viral video that had been circulating at the time: a video of about 20 cows crossing a country road, but jumping over the center white line of the road. The video was taken by a woman who isn't seen, but she is laughing throughout the 14-second clip. The news anchor laughed as the camera focused on him, saying, "Hahaha look at those cows! That's so funny. We'll be right back." I thought to myself, *That's fucking stupid*, and I changed the channel.

The next channel was a different news station. The anchor looked at the camera and said, "Hahaha look at those cows! That's so funny. We'll be right back." I looked closely at the TV.

That's odd, I thought. *They also showed the cows.*

I changed the channel. Next was some game show announcer who said, "Hahaha look at those cows! That's so funny. We'll be right back."

Weird! This video is on every channel?

I flipped to the next channel, the Spanish channel, Telemundo. Two people were standing on the set and in a Spanish accent said, "Hahaha look at those cows! That's so funny. We'll be right back."

"Holy shit," I stammered.

I turned off the TV and shook my head to try to get my thoughts in order. An MA came into the room and said, "Did you see those cows? That was so funny." I looked at her dumbfounded, mouth agape, probably looking terrified. She repeated, "I have to check your vital signs." I stammered, "Oh, yeah. Sure," as she wrapped the blood pressure cuff around my arm. She walked out of the room, and I sighed, "What the fuck is going on?"

I thought that if I watched something funny it would cheer me up and maybe fix whatever was happening in my head. I had been reading a biography of the American comic George Carlin, so I thought of one of his sketches, "Seven Words You Can Never Say on Television." I picked up my phone, slowly typed the title into YouTube, and clicked on the stand-up comedy routine from the early 1970's. If you have not seen Carlin's hilarious routine, please watch it now. If you have seen it, remember the seven words are: shit, piss, fuck, cunt, cocksucker, motherfucker, and tits. I watched the six-minute YouTube clip and laughed along. This hilarious routine had also succeeded in taking my mind off my circumstances. The clip ended and I chuckled as I put my phone down. I closed my eyes and lay my head on my pillow, trying not to mess up the wires protruding from my head. The seven words echoed in my head, and I continued to chuckle, but then different voices from the staff started to float into my room. They were all saying the foul words.

"Hi, Jim, how was your weekend?" a nurse asked her colleague.

"Well, you know, shit, piss, fuck, cunt, cocksucker, motherfucker, and tits," Jim replied.

WHAT DID HE SAY? I screamed in my head.

"Ok, Dr. Smith. How about the cocksucker, motherfucker in room 7?" a different voice asked.

"Well, he is getting better, but shit, piss, fuck, cunt," Dr. Smith replied.

OH MY GOD!

Then a small old woman working with a physical therapist walked down the hallway.

"How are you doing, Mrs. Jones?" asked the physical therapist.

"Well, shit, piss, fuck, cunt, cocksucker, motherfucker, and tits!" the old woman answered in a frail voice.

Holy shit. Now this has gotten even weirder.

In desperation, I covered my ears and tried to stop any voices coming in from the hallway. Although the profanity of the little old lady was remarkably hilarious, it was all the more terrifying. I half laughed and half cried at the absurdity of it all. I felt like I was doomed to descend into madness. Then a loud voice called out, "Mr. Celella, is everything alright?"

What the fuck? Who the fuck is that?

"Mr. Celella, can you hear me?"

Yes, I can hear you, I thought. My descent into madness just picked up speed. "Umm....Yes," I replied, "Yeah, I'm good...."

"Ok. We saw some spikes on your EEG. We were seeing if you had any seizures."

Ok, so this was the man behind the curtain! Now presenting himself as a voice emanating from the speakers overhead.

The video monitor and the EEG were linked to a central office, which was recording my every move and brain wave. They had seen me looking distraught and seen evidence of mini-seizures on the EEG. They could radio into my room and ask if I was ok. *Thanks, Big Brother.*

My father arrived a few minutes later. He asked me how I was doing. I told him I wasn't so good. A nurse came into the room as I recounted the previous few minutes. The cows, the seven words, the Big Brother control message. It took a long time to explain all the details, as I still had limited speech, often getting stuck and spouting obscenities. Then my wife called my father's phone and I could hear their conversation.

"How is he doing?" Caitlin asked my father.

"Well, some new developments this morning. Apparently, he's hearing voices."

"Cocksucker, motherfucker, tits!" exclaimed my wife, something she would never have said otherwise.

"Oh God, she is saying it, too!" I exclaimed.

"Wait. She is saying it, too?" my father asked while still on the phone with Caitlin.

"What are they doing to him?" Caitlin screamed in horror over the phone.

The echoes continued for 12 hilarious and horrifying hours. They mostly cycled around George Carlin's "Seven Words," but would usually stick to the last things the person in my room said. A nurse would say, "I'll see you later." I would hear, "I'll see you later, I'll see you later, I'll see you later, I'll see you later, I'll see you later, I'll see you later," multiple times from multiple different people out in the hallway. Then their speech would gradually return to the general vulgarity of George Carlin.

The medical term for this condition is "echolalia," defined as a meaningless repetition of another person's spoken words. This can be a symptom of a psychiatric disorder, autism, or head trauma. In my case, it was due to the seizures, both the three generalized seizures and the continued smaller seizures seen on EEG. The seizures were likely due to the bombardment of the chemo and radiation on the remaining tumor cells. As the tumor cells are destroyed by the chemo and radiation, they can cause inflammation, or swelling, of the brain which can trigger the onset of seizures. In addition, the cannabis and alcohol I was consuming increased the likelihood of having seizures. Add in the reaction to Dilantin with various anti-seizure medications, and I had multiple factors causing this echolalia.

That afternoon, the neurology team arrived to inform me that I was still having almost 25 mini seizures every hour. Of course, I had figured something was wrong, as George Carlin's words still reverberated in my head, yet I still didn't have the ability to express my thoughts in speech. My father had painstakingly pieced together my words in order to tell the neurology team about my echolalia. My anti-seizure medications were changed again. The Topamax was stopped and a nightly dose of 10 milligrams of Clobazam (Onfi) was started. Later that evening, the echolalia started to fade. I was able to get some better sleep.

Tuesday, August 27, 2019

I awoke to a wretched voice yelling, "I'm here to draw your blood and take your vitals!" All the lights turned on and pierced through my pupils. I shut my eyes only to see the bluish light swirl around my closed eyelids. A needle that felt as wide as a baseball bat plunged into my arm, wriggled back and forth, and then quickly withdrew. A Band-Aid was placed on the wound and a blood pressure cuff inflated over it. A sensor grabbed my finger, and a probe invaded my mouth. Everything withdrew and the voice said goodbye and turned off the light.

What the fuck just happened and where the fuck am I? I thought to myself.

It took me a few minutes to regain my bearings and remember the hell storm that had enveloped my life over the last few days. I turned on a softer light and sat up in bed, only to be reminded by the screeching alarm warning me not to sit up. I lay back and apologized to the Big Brother camera and the nursing staff. It took me about a half hour to get my head back on straight.

I was assisted to the bathroom and washed up. I got back into bed with the alarm armed. I didn't dare turn on the TV nor watch anything on my phone. I didn't want to hear any more voices, especially George Carlin. I heard normal voices out in the hallway. Fortunately, they were all normal and did not repeat. I breathed a deep sigh.

One of the residents from the neurological service walked into my room around 7:30 AM. I had seen her yesterday, and she asked me how I was feeling. I said I was a little better. My speech was starting to improve a bit. She quizzed me, asking me to name objects in the room. She pointed to her watch and asked what it was. I said, "Wh….watch." She held up a pen and I said, "pen." Then she pointed to the top clicker part of the pen and asked what it was. I said, "Fuck...a pen?" She laughed and said, "Ok." She told me that the seizures were slowing down and it seemed like the new meds were working. I would be seen by my oncologist and my radiation oncologist. Then the neurology team would come by later this afternoon. After a quick neuro exam, she left.

The day went slowly as I continued to have intermittent waves of echolalia. I was given a button to press if I had any seizure symptoms. If I heard repeating voices, I would press the button and a loud voice would call out, "Mr. Celella, are you ok?"

"Yes. I'm ok, just…fuck...just...hearing, fuck…hearing the repeating voices," I'd reply, as my own voice echoed in my head.

"Yes, we see a seizure spike here. Thank you," Big Brother would reply.

I would give a weary thumbs up and listen to the absurdity of what I'd just said. "Just hearing the voices again." One never expects to say that phrase to anyone in their lives.

My family was always by the side of my bed. Considering I could barely communicate with anyone, it was a blessing to have others to speak with the doctors and nurses. The day progressed, with my words returning slowly. I was having significantly less echolalia and gaining a much better command of my vocabulary. I was hoping that meant I was having fewer mini seizures.

I was seen by Matt Dodd, a physician's assistant who worked with Dr. Baehring. Given all the seizures, my chemotherapy regimen was on hold. As soon as the seizures were better controlled, I would restart the Temozolomide. Fortunately, Dr. Baehring is a trained neurologist with specialization in neuro-oncology, so he was on board and working closely with the neurology team in charge of my care during my stay in the hospital.

I was also seen by Leslie Long, a physician's assistant who worked with Dr. Contessa. My radiation treatments were also on hold because of my seizures. Ms. Long was a slight woman with a sorrowful gaze. I told her, "Never, never be up...fuck...on this side of the bed. It is terrible. Make sure you dig...fuck...die of a tragic accident and never have to be admitted to the hospital." I was frustrated and tired. I was generally cold and would interrupt her while she tried to explain when they would restart radiation.

"Once you're cleared by the neuro service, we will set up your radiation treatments," she softly started.

"Ok, so you have no idea when I'll start?" I interrupted.

"Well, once we hear from neuro, we'll let you know."

"Fine. Whatever," I coldly retorted.

In retrospect, I felt bad taking my anger out on Ms. Long. I was finally starting to get some words back, and had only used them to belittle her. She gracefully took my abuse and told me she would let me know when she heard from the neurology service.

Later that evening, the neurology service came and confirmed my suspicion that I was in fact having less seizure activity; however, the seizures were continuing. They increased my Clobazam (Onfi) to 15 milligrams nightly to see if that would help. If fewer seizures occurred, they would take the EEG off and restart my chemo and radiation.

I took more pills and hoped it would show improvement so I could get the EEG off and restart my cancer treatment. I wanted to plow through those treatments and finish them quickly.

Wednesday, August 28, 2019

Hospital day five started with another harsh awakening. I felt better from the start. I knew I was exhausted from tolerating hospital life, and now I had some hope the EEG would be removed. I didn't eat breakfast, expecting to restart my chemo pill regimen that morning.

The whole neurology service rounded around 9 AM, much earlier than usual. They told me that I was still having seizures overnight, but there were far fewer, and they would again increase the Clobazam (Onfi) to 20 milligrams nightly. However, I was going to get the EEG off and could resume my chemo and radiation. I quickly asked when I could go home, but I was met with resistance. The neurology team wanted to introduce the chemo and radiation and make sure I was seizure-free prior to discharge. This was not an unreasonable request; in fact, it was a good clinical judgment call. But at the time, I did not see it that way. All I wanted to do was go home.

So what if I could barely speak and couldn't read?! I could sit at home and do nothing that required reading, writing, or speaking, I thought.

I wanted to get the fuck out of that hospital. Attached to wires, the EEG, getting blood drawn every day and getting woken up at all hours of the night is not a pleasant state to live in.

I took my chemo pills and now 2000 milligrams of Keppra. Waited an hour and had some breakfast. Matt Dodd, the PA, came to visit and asked if I had any questions. I did not. I told him, "I'll see you after I get out of this hell hole." He smiled and agreed to meet me as an outpatient.

I was scheduled to go to my radiation treatment later that afternoon instead of my usual 9 AM appointment. I also saw Ms. Long. I apologized for my attitude and behavior the day before. She looked at me and went to shut the door. She came back and explained that she usually didn't tell people this, but, "Five years ago, I lost my husband to a glioblastoma. So I know how you and your wife are feeling, and how it is on your side of the bed. It is terrible. He had a different type of glioma, and you will likely survive for a long time." I was shocked. I stammered another apology and thanked her for sharing her story. She smiled her sorrowful smile and wished me the best of luck.

That afternoon, I was wheeled down to the radiation suite. I met with Dr. Contessa prior to receiving my radiation treatment. I asked why I hadn't been given Decadron or any other steroids to help slow the seizures and maybe help prevent them altogether. His reply was that if I had gotten the steroids, it might have helped the seizures, but it could also shrink the area where the radiation was targeting, causing the radiation to fire around the sides of the remaining tumor and hit other healthy tissue. The steroids could have altered the map they were using for radiation, rendering the treatments less effective and even damaging healthy brain cells. I told him I was glad they were not firing into the "good" part of my brain, then got through the session without any issues.

When I was wheeled back to the Epilepsy Unit, I was informed that I would be transferred off that floor to the general neurology floor, EP 7-7. I proceeded to make a huge stink about getting wheelchair transport.

"I'm going to get a fucking DVT (blood clot) if I can't walk around here. I'm walking, we're taking the stairs, no fucking wheelchair," I told the nursing staff. I don't know if it was out of pity, necessity, or they were just fed up with me, but they agreed to my demands. I walked to EP 7-7 and instantly recognized that it was the same floor I had been on two months earlier during my initial presentation and surgery.

It was around 5 PM when I arrived. The two nurses who walked me to the floor wished me good luck and returned to the epilepsy floor. I looked around my new room. There was an empty bed across the room and I looked up to see a "Fall Risk" sign on my door. This meant that I would still be on a bed alarm and would need help to go to the bathroom. I grabbed the sign and threw it away. Fortunately, no one seemed to notice.

My father and I sat and passed the time playing cards. Caitlin joined later that evening. I was hoping to have a good night's sleep and get discharged in the morning. I continued to have better control of my speech and finally felt like things were moving in a better direction.

Thursday, August 29, 2019

I awoke groggy. Six nights of interrupted sleep made it difficult to get any real rest. I met my nurse for the day, a sweet Asian woman who seemed like she had been working in medicine for a long time. She had been my nurse earlier that summer. She was no-nonsense, but had a twinkle of mischief in her eyes. She was nice enough to treat me less like a prisoner and more like an educated healthcare provider.

I had already been up and about around the room. On the wall there was a whiteboard with a variety of information, such as nurses and MA names, day and room number, kitchen number for food, and pain score. I had slowly and painstakingly written my idea of the day's schedule:

7 AM-chemo

8 AM-breakfast

9 AM-radiation

10 AM-meet with neuro team

11 AM-discharge or leave AMA (against medical advice)

My nurse laughed at the AMA bullet point on the whiteboard. In a half joking, half serious tone I told her that I would certainly be leaving today. She agreed, both happy to get rid of me and also wishing me well.

The neurology resident came by and asked me some different questions to assess my neurological status. My speech was better and my recall of familiar ideas was improving. I was far from 100%, but was saying "fuck" a little less and was able to have a slow conversation. I was still virtually unable to read; only at a painstakingly slow pace and with lots of re-reading the text was I able to comprehend the words. The resident said that I would be discharged later that morning as long as I had no seizures during the radiation and chemo.

I took my chemo. I took my Keppra and had some breakfast. However, I did not get a cup of coffee with my breakfast tray. I was already in my street clothes, sporting a Yale shirt, and thought a nice little walk to get some coffee would help my physique. I casually walked to the unit secretary and quickly announced, "I'm just going to run down and grab a coffee. I'll be right back," as I slipped out the door to the elevators.

I got to the bottom floor and headed to one of the many coffee stations. Then I froze.

Shit! I don't have my wallet or any money.

I then chose a coffee station that was near a quick hallway exit, one mostly used by staff. I filled up a cup of coffee, and moving quickly and acting like I was missing an important meeting, slipped out the door into the hallway. As I looked back to see if anyone had seen, I made eye contact with the neurology resident that had come to assess me earlier that morning. I quickly took out my cell phone and looked away. She didn't seem to notice or did not want to notice. Obviously, I don't condone stealing, but at the time I rationalized that my insurance and I had given the hospital close to a million dollars over the last two months, and that I still owed about $100,000 to Yale for my education. The Yale Business Machine could spare a $1.50 cup of coffee.

I returned to the floor. The door was locked and I had to press the buzzer to be let in. A voice chattered, "Yes, can I help you?"

"Yes, I need to get back in," I answered.

"Who is the patient?"

"Uhh, me."

The door opened. The secretary was not happy. "Oh my god! I didn't realize you were the patient when you left!"

"I was only gone for a few minutes."

"You're going to get me into trouble, Mr. Celella."

"No, no. I wouldn't dream of that. I'll be in more trouble than you will!"

My nurse with the twinkle of mischief laughed when I recounted my adventure. She sighed and said, "I'm always sad to see the nice patients leave."

Miraculously, I was wheeled down to my radiation appointment right on time. I completed the treatment without any issue. I was wheeled back up to the room. Caitlin was waiting for me.

The neurology team rounded around 10:30 AM and agreed that I could be discharged. I was sent home on a veritable truckload of anti-seizure prescriptions: 2000 milligrams of Keppra in the morning and at night with 20 milligrams of Onfi at night. The Keppra pills are huge white horse pills in 1000 milligram formulations, meaning I would take two in the morning and two at night. 4000 milligrams every day. The Onfi are small, white, bitter little pills that turn your mouth dry and sour. We were instructed to watch out for seizures, and if I had one, whoever was with me should time the seizure and wait until I woke up and spoke. If I didn't have any more seizures after that, I could stay home. If I continued to have seizures or did not come out of a postictal state, that would constitute an emergency. This was hardly welcome advice to my wife, who had now seen me seize at least five times, no doubt giving her some form of PTSD.

When I got home, I threw away all the cannabis products in the house. The feeling of getting high and then progressing to seizure was too much to ever use cannabis again. That day, I also swore off alcohol forever. Knowing that it lowers my seizure threshold, not to mention its litany of toxic effects, was enough never to drink again. As an avid beer and whiskey connoisseur and ambitious homebrewer, I thought it would be hard to stop drinking alcohol. However, after the loss of my speech, writing, and reading, it was surprisingly easy to put the bottle down.

I figured the cessation of my bad habits and addition of new anti-seizure drugs would lead to an easy recovery from this hospital stay, just as after the brain surgery. But this was only the beginning of a hellish descent into madness over the next months. First, the nightmares started.

65-year-old male with brain tumor

I was working at a Connecticut hospital when a 65-year-old Hispanic male with a past medical history of coronary artery disease and diabetes came into the hospital with altered mental status. The CT scan showed a large 4 cm left frontal mass. He did recall his name and his date of birth, but could not remember the events leading to his arrival in the ER. I was called to admit him to the hospitalist service given his altered mental status, which was complicated by a urinary tract infection in the diabetic male. I asked the ER physician if he had told the patient about the large mass; the physician replied that he had not told the patient because the man was primarily Spanish-speaking. This job was left to me.

Unfortunately, the language barrier necessitated a telephone translation service. Essentially, the system had two telephone receivers, one for me and one for the patient. A Spanish language interpreter spoke to both of us through these two telephone receivers. I had to tell the patient and his wife, sitting closely at the bedside, that he had to be brought into the hospital because of the mass on his brain. I can still remember him sobbing with his wife, who was virtually inconsolable, while I tried to explain the specifics of how we would also work up this brain mass and treat his urinary tract infection.

I was trying to convey the seriousness of this information, but with the limitations of the telephone translation service, they were extremely difficult to impart to the patient and his wife. Their sobs continue to haunt me as I can still see their faces after they heard the words "brain mass."

It is important to note how in medicine, especially diagnostic imaging, we use the term "mass" when explaining to patients the seriousness of their condition. On imaging, radiologists cannot tell precisely if a mass is a tumor, malignant or benign, if it is new or old, or has been there the patient's entire life. All you can see is that there is something. In order to find out if the mass is in fact malignant or benign, one needs to complete a biopsy. If it had been an intracranial bleed, this would've been quite clear on the CT scan. MRIs can provide additional information and can better categorize what type of mass is present. Ultimately, the best way to determine the mass' diagnosis is through biopsy reports, tumor markers, DNA analysis, and putting slides under a microscope.

While it's difficult to explain the above information through a translator to someone without medical training, it's virtually impossible to do so while that person is deep in the throes of grief, sorrow, and profound loss.

58-year-old female with blown pupil

Late one evening, I admitted a very friendly 58-year-old female with a severe urinary tract infection. She had come to the ER with fever and low back pain. She had a CT scan of her abdomen, which showed some hydronephrosis and fluid around her kidneys. Usually this is a sign of pyelonephritis, or kidney infection. After reviewing the CT scan, bloodwork, vital signs, and her insignificant medical history, I went to examine her and explain that she would be admitted to the hospital. I did a quick exam, listening to her heart, lungs, and belly, paying particular attention to her lower back, where the kidneys are located. I admitted her to the general medical floor with IV antibiotics, IV fluids, and antipyretics (anti-fever meds, like Tylenol).

I went about writing the admission history and physical note. The nature of her admission is a very common diagnosis. Considering she had no other medical problems, it was a very straightforward admission. I figured she would likely improve within a few days and could be discharged home.

I got a call from the RN who was receiving her on the medical floor. While getting the patient into the hospital bed and completing her own physical exam, she noticed the patient's left pupil was slightly larger than the right. If the difference of pupil size is small, it may be a normal variant, especially if the patient is asymptomatic. However, in other cases it could indicate a neurological or ophthalmological emergency. I went back to see the patient. Indeed, she did have the faintest difference in pupil dilation. She denied any other symptoms and said she had never noticed it before. I sort of shrugged, but ordered a CT of her head to be absolutely certain nothing was abnormal.

My jaw dropped at the scan. Essentially, the entire left side of her brain was a massive tumor. It was pushing on her right side and down into her left eye, causing her small pupil defect.

Friday, August 30-Monday, September 1, 2019

I finally arrived home and was greeted by my two boys screaming with joy at seeing me again. Their cheers of "Dada's home!" were both endearing to my heart and damning to my ears. Since the seizures, my sensitivity to high-pitched sounds had become much worse. My pounding headaches became more constant, now accompanied by nausea. I felt perpetually hungover, but without any of the fun of getting drunk.

That night I took my four pills (two Keppra, two Onfi) and went happily to my own bed. I fell asleep as soon as I hit the pillow, but then slept restlessly. I woke up several times with cold sweats. I was having incredibly vivid dreams. Some of them centered around being trapped in an exam room or tied to a stretcher. I would get bad news about my diagnosis or be forced into nonconsensual operations or procedures.

Other times, the nightmares would focus on patients I had treated in the past who had died.

A kind woman in her 40s who had come in with fevers and wound up having advanced liver cancer that had metastasized throughout her whole body, and died a few days later.

A man in his 70s whom I cared for every time he was admitted to the hospital for IV chemo treatments. He died three years after I first met him.

A woman in her 50s who was in the hospital for a UTI, but found one of her pupils was larger than the other. She had an enormous glioblastoma and died within a week of diagnosis.

Another woman, 42 years old and frail, who was walking and suddenly broke her leg. She had advanced bone cancer and died in hospice. I pronounced her dead and had to tell her husband and two children, ages ten and eight, that they would never see their mom again.

Dozens of souls would come to visit me in my dreams. Some angry, some sorrowful, some indifferent. The dreams were punctuated by the Hispanic man sobbing uncontrollably after I'd told him he had a brain mass.

By far the worst were the memories of children I'd treated. During my days on the ambulance and while working at Tufts Medical Center (which had a level 1 pediatric trauma center), I had seen a handful of children die. Two shaken baby syndromes, one SIDS patient, a 5-year-old and an 8-year-old who were hit by cars, and a 16-year-old who died from bacterial meningitis. These children would appear in different places in my dreams, but frequently they would be on a playground, all on a merry-go-round with the 16-year-old girl pushing them. An eerie "Ring around the Rosie" tune would start and fade into the same uncontrollable sobbing from the Hispanic man with the brain mass. I would shoot up out of bed gasping for air and dripping with sweat.

The nightmares got more vivid and intense the further along I got in my chemo and radiation courses. Towards the end of the initial treatments, at the end of September, I was becoming afraid to sleep. I would lie in bed and try to keep my eyes open as long as I could so I wouldn't have to face all the demons in my dreams. I was napping during the afternoons when my children did, but those souls were waiting for me, even in the daylight.

My poor wife had it worse. Vinny was not a very good sleeper and would often have tooth pain or gas or just be generally needy at night. He would wake screaming in his room, and she would run over and comfort him while I slept. Then she would hear me wake up gasping for breath and moving suddenly; she would leave our son, run to our bedroom to make sure I wasn't seizing, then run back to my son to make sure he didn't fall out of bed. No one in my house got much rest.

When I was discharged from my seizure admission on August 29th, I knew that I had to be back at the hospital the next day for radiation treatment. Like going back to prison as a free man. The radiation continued without any seizures, but the effects began to build. First were the increasing headaches. They would be pounding and unceasing. A mechanized hammer drilling constantly in my head. No drugs would help. I tried every over-the-counter remedy with no relief. My oncologist and radiologist offered migraine medications, which I refused, given potential interactions with my seizure meds. They also offered low-dose opioids, which I also refused, because I didn't want to start down any path with opioids. I also didn't want any other medication that would cause more disruption of my brain function. I reasoned that after the chemo and radiation assault on my brain was over, things would start to get better, so I could tough it out for a few more months.

Then the sensitivity to blue light increased tenfold. The radiation machine had a guide laser that would cross my field of vision three times. Despite my eyes being closed, I could see it through my eyelids. This blue was accompanied by an acrid taste like burning wires. After my treatments, I would see the blue lights flicker on my field of vision. Then if I saw the bright sun, or any other blue light, it would cause me to have the same acrid taste. Anything I ate would turn to ash in my mouth. At night, blue lights from police cars were especially brutal. While watching TV, any police car, welding metal, sparks flying, or fireworks would set off that acrid taste. It would last for two to three hours every time I saw a bright blue light. Most of the day and night I felt as if I had ash in my mouth, and I really didn't eat much.

The sensitivity to sound was exponentially worse. High-pitched noises would cascade through my head like ice picks. With my two young sons, I was in for a lot of screaming and high-pitched noises. Clinking glasses or silverware at restaurants was a nightmare. I always carried earplugs and had to wear them almost all the time. I could not even stand to be near my children nor most of my large Italian family because the noise would be too much for my head. My older son, only two-and-a-half years old, would see me wince if he yelled or something fell in the kitchen. He would say, "I'm sorry your brain hurts," as I yelled in frustration multiple times a day, "That [sound, yell, something] is hurting my brain!"

The nausea never led to vomiting, but was more like a constant gnawing of half hunger pains and half disgust at eating. Ads on TV with huge burgers or pizza would make me cringe. When my messy toddlers ate, I would have to look away from their pasta sauce-covered hands and faces. This was on top of the acrid taste that was almost always present. I would eat a small piece of peanut butter toast in the morning with a cup of coffee. Usually skip lunch, as I would have just come home from radiation with the acrid taste and then watched my children eat the way toddlers do—like savage, drunk racoons. Then the minute I felt hungry I would try to eat anything I could. But I would feel so full so fast that I ended up eating only a few bits of what I had prepared.

All of these symptoms: the nightmares, headaches, light and sound sensitivity, and nausea just got progressively worse as the chemo and radiation treatments continued.

October 2019

October started with the huge accomplishment of finishing radiation. I shook hands and thanked many people. In the waiting room next to the giant fish tank was a large gong. When patients finish their radiation regimens, they swing the hammer and ring the gong. Patients' family and friends would come and take pictures and weep with tears of joy. Caitlin, my uncle Kevin, and cousin Mitchell came to help me celebrate. I swung the hammer and rang out a loud crash, as if the emperor himself was in the front of the waiting room. It was a moment of brief happiness.

As a parting gift, I was given the radiation mask that had been molded to my face. I thought for sure that I was going to ax it to pieces when I got home, but it is still tucked away in my garage. I'm not sure what I will do with it, and am wondering if it is emitting a bunch of radiation. Yet it was nice to take it off the shelf at YNHH and know I would not be needing it anymore.

By the end of the first round of six weeks of chemo on September 26th and the end of radiation on October 1st, I had lost 30 pounds, wore earplugs all the time, had an acrid taste permanently in my mouth, barely ate, couldn't sleep, and was losing hope.

After finishing my radiation and first round of chemo, I had the whole month of October "off." No further chemo or radiation. I would wait one month for any swelling to subside and then get an MRI on November 1st to evaluate the progress. About halfway through October, I started to feel a little better. I continued my afternoon naps but still had nightmares. Although waning, my other symptoms of constant headaches and light and sound sensitivity continued. The nausea waned but was replaced by early satiety, or feeling full after small meals. Prior to the surgery I had been a big eater, able to clean off plates and plates of food. I had radically changed my diet both out of necessity and also to try anything that may help stop the cancer from growing. Instead of eating two giant helpings of pasta and processed foods, I was only able to eat a small salad with half a piece of chicken, much to the chagrin of my Italian grandmother, who saw cooking and eating as happiness.

Since the end of August, I had been virtually unable to read. Gradually, it returned to where I was able to slowly read a text message and type a reply. Ralphie, my two-and-a-half-year-old son, was an avid reader, and I wasn't able to read quickly or smoothly enough to keep him engaged. Although he couldn't read, he had memorized most of his books and would often correct me when I said something wrong. I remember reading "Goodnight Moon," by Margaret Wise Brown, and taking a long time to read the words, "Three little breads sitting on chairs," only to be interrupted by him, "No, Daddy! It says 'bears,' not 'breads!'"

This is true humility and shame, when your toddler can read better than you after you've received an Ivy League education.

After finishing radiation, my reading started to improve. While Ralphie napped, I would grab his books off the shelf and go through them page by page, pick out words that I could not recognize, and start writing them out, by hand, five times each. "The cow that jumped over the moon," was written vertically:

The cow that jumped over the moon
The cow that jumped over the moon
The cow that jumped over the moon
The cow that jumped over the moon
The cow that jumped over the moon

I would count this as my "physical therapy." Over the month of October, I filled two small notebooks of words. Certain word families would cause me big problems, such as words starting with "wh" (where, when, what, which), "th" (there, their, threw, though, through, thought). Words beginning with the following prefixes were especially difficult: inter-, com-, sh-, and ch-. Also, it was common for me to switch similar sounding letters, like F and V, P and B, B and D.

Interestingly, when I was a child in elementary school, I'd had similar issues with spelling and recognizing some of these same words. I may have had a mild form of dyslexia. Over the years, I'd just found ways to work around it, and had obviously overcome the issues in order to get an advanced education. Now I felt like a neurological connection had been severed during my brain surgery and exacerbated by the seizures, radiation, and chemo, and I had to start finding new ways to learn how to read.

My son seemed less impressed and would bring me books with few words, adding, "Here, Dad. This is an easy book for you."

"Thanks for the encouragement, Ralphie." Apparently, toddlers don't understand sarcasm.

While I was rehabbing my reading skills, I tried to restart some of my usual hobbies and coping mechanisms. However, most of my coping mechanisms had been stripped away from me like my reading. I ran three marathons in college, but stopped running while in grad school. I was just starting to get back into it, and had run five miles the morning of my first seizure in June. I couldn't run during treatment, as my headaches were getting progressively worse.

I loved to drive. Getting in the car and just going somewhere—or nowhere—and getting a sense of the open road always put my mind at ease. I had traveled cross country after college, stopping at 16 national parks, and covering all but five states in the USA (the five I haven't been to are: Nebraska, North Dakota, Kentucky, Kansas, and Hawaii). But then I couldn't drive. In Connecticut, you are forbidden to drive until being seizure-free for three months. After the seizures in August, I couldn't drive myself around. I would have to wait until the end of November.

I had learned how to cook from my Italian grandmother. I was able to gather anything from a pantry and create a meal; I consider myself a fairly good cook. I love to put together a big meal and share it with my family. I would try new recipes and also cook for my wife—who barely cooks at all—and the children. A glass of beer would often accompany me in the kitchen, as my homebrewing was continuous. Churning out about five gallons of beer every month, and sharing it with many friends, I also drank a hefty portion myself. Now I barely could eat. Nausea would envelop me when I smelled food, watching the kids eat was horrifying, and the acrid taste left by radiation treatments put me off most foods. I couldn't and also didn't want to drink alcohol, and so my homebrew equipment collected dust.

One of my only coping mechanisms left was singing. I had been singing in academic choirs since middle school. I'm a fairly good first tenor with a wide vocal range, well into the bass section. I can read music well and am a decent sight reader. I am trained classically, but without advanced degrees, only lengthy experience. In college, I sang with the Northeastern University choirs and chamber chorus, performing choral classics like Handel's "Messiah," Bach's "B Minor Mass," Carl Orff's "Carmina Burana," and Beethoven's "9th Symphony."

I developed into a classical music junkie, attending concerts at Symphony Hall and local churches. I would find many free concerts of Berklee College of Music and New England Conservatory students playing master's recitals. When I returned home to Connecticut and started at Yale School of Nursing, I auditioned for the Yale Camerata, a graduate and professional choir directed by Maggie Brooks. This placed me into a large community of singers who are far more talented than I am. We would perform regularly at Woolsey Hall with the Yale Glee Club, Yale Philharmonia, and

Yale Symphony. I've even made an appearance singing in Carnegie Hall with Caitlin and our St. Peter's Church choir. We were part of a large choir singing "Sancta Civitas," by Ralph Vaughan Williams.

Even though I had missed my yearly audition due to the seizures, I started up with the Yale Camerata for my fifth year in early September 2019. It was a bright shimmer of hope in a dark time. I got out of the house for a few hours on Tuesday nights to sing with some of the most talented musicians in the area. Maggie Brooks, the conductor of the group, was part of the Yale Institute of Sacred Music and also the head of the Master's in Choral Conducting program. Six conducting students would learn to hone their craft in front of the 80-voice choir.

The choir is made up of Yale graduate students who are studying a variety of disciplines, such as medicine, art, music, science, literature, and other academic pursuits. In addition to young grad students were local professionals: Yale faculty and staff, architects, lawyers, doctors, teachers, and musicians. It is a powerful experience to unite with people from all different backgrounds and specialties to make music together.

At the start of rehearsals, I could still barely read. It would take me a veritable eternity to get through the first sentence of the welcome letter from Maggie. However, I had no trouble following the musical notes. I could read the musical notations, sing the correct pitches and intervals, and all in time, but as soon as I had to sing with words, I would slip up. Thankfully, we had an assortment of languages in our repertoire, from Russian to German, Italian, and Spanish. When I sang in other languages, I had no problem keeping up with the text, because I didn't have to process the words I was saying. I merely had to use my voice to sing foreign text and the notes. It's funny how my right-sided brain was working with singing and producing other languages, while my left brain—bombarded by chemo and radiation—couldn't keep up with the reading.

Coincidences

Beginning in September, I started noticing a strange set of circumstances and situations which seemed like the plot of a conspiracy theory. Little farcical twists that could be strung into proof of existence of a higher being or simply coincidences that only the bored would notice.

One of the pieces the Yale Camerata would sing in our October concert was "A Procession Winding Around Me," for SATB choir with guitar accompaniment and music by Jeffrey Van. The piece was set to a collection of poems by Walt Whitman. The poems were: "By the Bivouac's Fitful Flame," "Beat! Beat! Drums!," "Look Down Fair Moon," and "Reconciliation." These were some of the poems written by Whitman during the Civil War, and also the same poems used in Ralph Vaughan Williams' piece "Dona Nobis Pacem." The text of "Reconciliation" was the same I had sung during my brain operation. I was shocked to see it slated for the October concert. Stunned, as I had no trouble singing these words, albeit set to different music. Jeffrey Van's piece is softer than Vaughan Williams'; it is more tender and has a more diverse eight-part harmony. Performing this same text now in Battell Chapel, instead of the OR with scalpels in my brain, was cathartic and chilling.

October was a renewal. While the leaves showed brilliant reds, yellows, and oranges, my mind and body had a miniature spring. Since ending chemo in late September and ringing the gong, signifying the end of radiation on October 1st, I felt better and better every day. My wife and I celebrated our eighth wedding anniversary on October 8th. I continued taking my afternoon naps, but started to shorten them. Some of my symptoms were resolving, but headaches continued.

I would often joke about getting a superpower after the surgery. Would I be like a stereotypical comic book character who gains some superpower after a traumatic event? Like how Peter Parker was bitten by a spider and then became Spider Man. I was half joking with many people that I was waiting for my power to be bestowed; nothing really materialized. However, I did start to recognize many people I saw in public. I had this overwhelming feeling that I knew them from somewhere. Just walking in the park or the grocery store, for most people I saw, I would think, "Where do I know them from?" I think it was a combination of the seizures and the anti-seizure medications, or possibly the nightmares, or just the thousands of people I have treated over my career in medicine. To this day, I will look at people and feel like I have had some interaction with them at some time in my life.

In October, my good friend Justin was divorcing his wife. They had been married two years earlier. I had been the officiant at his wedding and felt somewhat responsible for his marriage ending. He needed to sell his house, which was about a mile from mine. During my month break from treatment, I would walk up the road to his house and complete little construction projects while he was at work. It got me away from the kids and gave me something to do. I repainted most of the interior of his house to get it ready for sale. I used his stereo system to quietly play classical music, sometimes singing along with pieces I knew, sometimes sitting and crying between paint brush strokes. Familiar tunes would sway my moods, some happy, some sad, most reminiscent of a different time before all the brain cancer. Justin and I shared a bond of grief, me with a cancer diagnosis and him with his divorce. He would drive me to Camerata rehearsals and I would continue to paint his house. It was an even trade. He sold the house in December. It's funny how friends can have similar battles on different fields.

As October waned, I realized that my APRN license was set to expire in July of 2020. I had to start getting together a large number of continuing medical education (CME) credits as part of the re-licensure process. A three-day course called Update in Hospital Medicine 2019, presented by Harvard Medical School, fit the bill. It would run from Monday, October 28th to Wednesday, October 30th and give me almost half of the CME credits I needed for re-licensure. I thought it would be a perfect opportunity to review my medical knowledge and challenge me to see if I could keep up. I got the courses in book form and was able to take notes and follow along with the presenters.

The conference was held at the Copley Marriott in the center of Boston, only a few blocks from my alma mater, Northeastern University. I knew the area well and loved the city I'd called home for four years. Caitlin came with me, and my parents took care of the kids for the few days we were gone. The time in Boston also allowed us to see friends and family in the area. Being avid Boston sports fans, we made sure to catch a Boston Bruins hockey game.

The Bruins played the San Jose Sharks one night. As it was a Tuesday night game, we got great seats—about ten rows back from center ice. Caitlin went for a tour of TD Garden, the Bruins' home ice, on the day of the game—I was at the conference—and she returned with news of a strange coincidence. This game would be "Hockey Fights Cancer" night. That was all the preparation we would get, as we'd had no idea this was "Hockey Fights Cancer" night.

At the entrances to the arena there were posters available with a purple heading reading, "I Fight For" with a white space for fans to write in someone who had been affected by cancer. We walked past the first couple of tables, all stacked high with signs. I took a few minutes to decide if I wanted to present my current fight in this public area; Caitlin followed my lead and waited to see if I'd make a sign. I finally found a table, took a sign, and wrote, "I Fight For: MY BRAIN." Caitlin wrote, "HIS BRAIN." We held up our signs when prompted during the first intermission, which was a moving minute for us. The guy sitting next to me glanced at my sign and asked me how I was doing. Then he revealed that he'd fought cancer once already, and was looking down the barrel of another surgery in a couple weeks. Everyone was fighting their own battle. Thankfully, the Bruins won 1-5. There were three fights, almost 100 minutes of penalties served, five solid goals, and 17,000 screaming fans. The rout of the Sharks paired with the intense battles and favorable outcome felt like a good omen.

Prior to leaving for the trip to Boston, I scheduled an MRI for November 1st, 2019. I made the call while sitting on my deck looking out at a large dead ash tree at the edge of the woods. If I got bad news from the MRI, I was going to get my ax and hack that dead tree down bit by bit. No matter the headaches, pain, or even if I accidently plunged the ax into my foot, that dead tree would take the brunt of my grief and anger and come crashing down. Every time I went out to the deck or passed the window, I would stare at that dead tree, angrily plotting where I would swing the ax first. I would fixate my anger on that tree. When we came home from Boston on October 31st, I looked out the window, and the tree was gone. I was puzzled at first. Was I looking in the wrong spot? Was I sure it was actually gone? Through the window, I couldn't see if it had merely fallen down because it was then covered by a large number of thorns and overgrowth. I had to wait until the next morning to go and see where it had gone.

Friday, November 1, 2019

The next day was All Saints' Day. I took the dog out that morning and walked behind our house and into the woods. The tree I'd marked for death had been uprooted and fallen into the underbrush. I slowly turned and walked back to the house, befuddled that the tree which I'd wanted to fell had already fallen. There had been a lot of wind and rain that weekend, and presumably the elements had caused the tree to fall. I didn't know what to think, and was basically silent, busy pondering the meaning of this felled, deceased ash tree, until my MRI at 9:00 that morning.

My mother and grandmother came to watch the children while Caitlin and I went to the appointments. I was still pondering the meaning of the fallen tree while latent anxiety crept through me. *Would the MRI show improvement? Would it show increasing cancer? No effect of the radiation and chemo? Was it all for naught?*

These questions circled around my pounding head as my heart fluttered with trepidation. I got to the MRI department at YNHH, an off-site facility in a small basement clinic across the street. This was the first MRI after July, before chemo and radiation. I was handed a hospital gown, changed, and moved to the MRI suite. I lay on the table and the sheath was placed onto my face. The standard MRI sheath for my head was remarkably wider than the fitted radiation hood. Just lying on the table and having so much room around my face brought a sigh of relief.

I closed my eyes as the table moved me into position under the MRI. The machine roared to life. The clicks, bangs, and shaking started rumbling. I tried to make myself think of all the cancer cells that had died; it would be gone. I thought of how I had felt under the radiation machine, imagining the artillery fire and the fierce fighting of the chemo that I had struggled through over those seven weeks. I was "willing" my scan to look good, although deep down, I felt like it was too late, like I had already waged the battles, and now I was left to count the dead.

The voice of the MRI technician beeped overhead, "Ok, we're going to inject the contrast now." I was ripped out of my own thoughts. I said, "Ok. Sounds good," while trying to remember what I had been thinking about. The warmth of the contrast rushed through me, followed by the familiar metallic taste in my mouth. The clicks, bangs, and shaking of the machine restarted. About 15 minutes later, the scan was complete. The complete scan—brain MRI with and without contrast—takes about 45 minutes. Then I was off the table, given back my clothes, and we walked across the street to the formidable Smilow Cancer Hospital.

Caitlin and I went up the elevators to the eighth floor. The wait was on. We sat next to the fish tank; thankfully there were no dead fish in the tank. I was taken in for my vitals and placed in the Solarium, again appreciating the sick irony of "The World's Most Difficult Jigsaw Puzzle." After what seemed like an eternity, we were ushered into the same exam room where I was first told about the biopsy reports. A tall African American woman knocked on the door and introduced herself. Even before she finished, I asked to just see Dr. Baehring. Caitlin and I had agreed that on this occasion we wanted to hear the MRI results from the attending physician himself, and not one of his lackeys. We briefly told the woman of the previous negative experience, apologized, and asked to see Dr. Baehring. She gracefully acquiesced and left the room.

Dr. Baehring arrived a little later. He sternly said hello, sat, and got right to business. He opened the MRI pictures and showed me the results. I breathed a long sigh of relief. I knew that there was significant improvement before he said anything. We reviewed the scans and were so happy with the result: a significant amount of the residual tumor was now gone. All the pain, surgery, chemo, radiation, headaches, nausea, and suffering had been worth it!

I apologized to Dr. Baehring again for kicking the resident out of the room earlier. I know what it's like to go and see a patient and not have all the answers, then have to go back and write notes and present the patient's chart to the attending. It's a lot of work for the residents, and it's the way they learn how to become competent physicians. I suppose I made her day by not being someone she had to write a note about. Dr. Baehring cracked a small smile, which I had never seen before. He told me not to worry about it.

We discussed the next six chemo cycles. The dose of chemo would double, from 155 mg to 310 mg. If I tolerated that dose, it would be increased another 25% to 385 mg for the remaining five cycles. The schedule would be to take the Temozolomide for five days, then off for 23 days, which completes a 28-day cycle. The chemo pills would be hard at work killing cancer cells for that whole period, even though I'd only take the pills for five days each cycle.

Blood work, called a complete blood count (CBC) and comprehensive metabolic panel (CMP), would check my blood counts, immune system function, electrolytes, and kidney and liver function. I would get blood work on day 21 and 27 of the cycles, as this would be my nadir. A nadir is the term for the lowest point of immune system function, usually on day 21. Then the day 27 blood work would ensure my immune system function was starting to recover, and I could start the next cycle.

I felt ready for anything after hearing the good news of the MRI. I quickly agreed to the next cycles and waited to start. We left the hospital feeling elated for the first time in months.

That Sunday, in celebration of All Saints' Day, we sang a wonderful hymn at St. Peter's, "For All the Saints," a classic processional for an All Saints' service. The tune of the hymn is called "Sine Nomine," or "Without Name." It was composed by none other than Ralph Vaughan Williams. Chills shot through me as I sang another one of his pieces, another beautiful coincidence. The words of the hymn were written by William Walsham How, a 19th century English bishop, and they resonated with me through the stanza:

"But lo! there breaks a yet more glorious day;
the saints triumphant rise in bright array;
the King of glory passes on his way.
Alleluia, Alleluia!"

Wednesday, November 13, 2019

After my meeting with Dr. Baehring on November 1st, I was slated to start chemo again the next week. However, I had difficulty arranging the delivery of my medications. In order to receive my chemo meds, a long series of events had to take place. First, the Temozolomide had to be ordered by Dr. Baehring. That order was then transferred to the YNHH Pharmacy. The YNHH Pharmacy verified the order and processed it through Aetna, my insurance carrier. Aetna would deny the Temozolomide because its protocols stated this particular drug had to come from Aetna Specialty Pharmacy. The order was then transferred to Aetna Specialty Pharmacy. It was again verified and processed through my Aetna plan.

Then Aetna Specialty Pharmacy personnel called me to verify the order, confirmed that I understood how to take the medication, and answered any questions I had. I would pay any copays. Then they would arrange for UPS shipping, and the meds would be delivered a few days later. Then I had to call Dr. Baehring's office to again verify the drug, dosage, route, and time. They would give me the go ahead, and I would start the chemo the next day.

This truly dizzying and convoluted process would often get held up or stopped for some reason. Then I would have to call Dr. Baehring's office, YNHH Pharmacy, Aetna Specialty Pharmacy, or UPS to track down the stage of processing for the medication. During the first chemo cycle, I got to be on a first-name basis with all the individual players. Fortunately, because of my healthcare experience, I was able to get through to the right people. I knew who I needed to ask, who was worthless and couldn't help me, and who I could rely on to get things done. I almost always introduced myself as an APRN, so I got attention and respect from the people I spoke with. I did not take "no" for an answer, and I was not afraid to escalate my concerns, my profanity, or my advocacy. This would prove to be a recurring theme throughout my treatment.

After many phone calls, I received the Temozolomide and hoped that I wouldn't have to do all that work to get this med every cycle, as I would have to repeat the same amount of work every time. I started the chemo and it hit like a fucking train, plane, and meteor all at once.

I thought for sure it would be easy to get through the chemo without the burden of radiation, but the double dose of medication felt like 10 times more. My headaches were throbbing all the time with sharp spikes through the scar. Like a monkey with pots and pans bashing together in my head. Lights and noise were torture. Even switching on a soft light would send ice picks through my head. Just clinking a fork from the drawer would make me wince. The screams and loud noises of my toddlers were like nails on a chalkboard. The acrid taste was constant, making my mouth like ash, even while drinking water.

The nightmares got even more vivid. Now the tortured souls were looking at me and screaming, causing my head to feel pain in my dreams, only to spring awake to the reality of my living nightmare.

I didn't want to sleep, and I couldn't eat. I was miserable and bitter all month long. I continued to answer robocalls and scream obscenities to the chirping recorded voice telling me to get an extended warranty on my car.

Thanksgiving came. My in-laws came to stay with us, but would stand by helpless and worried for me and Caitlin. We had our Thanksgiving meal with my family and I could barely get down a bite of turkey. Then in a terrible twist of kicking me while I was down, I had to replace my kitchen faucet as it sprang a leak and spurted water all over the kitchen and basement. My chorus of "Shit!" and "Fuck!" echoed over Thanksgiving leftovers.

I saw Dr. Baehring's PA at the end of November and complained about the headaches. To illustrate my point, I took the computer mouse and banged it on the table while loudly talking to the PA. Apparently, it caused a commotion, as a few staff members came rushing into the exam room to ask if everything was OK. I told them that is what my head felt like all the time. The PA kindly offered more pills, either mild opioids or antimigraine medications. I refused. None of the over-the-counter meds worked. I didn't want to be some junky, nor start adding more meds to my impressive anti-seizure regimen.

The PA then offered a referral to a headache specialist. I laughed indignantly and said, "Yeah, I'll see them by the time I'm either dead or done with the chemo cycles." After some pressing from my wife and the PA, I reluctantly agreed. Sure enough, I got an

appointment at the Yale headache clinic on February 19, 2020—
nearly three months later.

I was so frustrated with the visit; I didn't say anything else and just
assured everyone I was fine. I didn't want to delve into any more of
my symptoms just to be offered different drugs, bullshit
appointments, or feigned empathy. I essentially stormed out and told
the PA to just order the next cycle of chemo and check the
obituaries.

A few days later, I started the whole process of tracking down my
chemo meds and getting them delivered. I called Dr. Baehring's
office, YNHH pharmacy, and Aetna Specialty Pharmacy. The hold
music was deafening, exacerbated by the screaming children. My
blood work looked good, and so the dose of Temozolomide was
increased another 25% to 385 mg. I would start the next cycle on
December 11th.

Wednesday, December 11, 2019

As I crossed into December, I started to feel marginally better. I gradually had fewer symptoms, but headaches were still gnawing through my brain. I was still singing, albeit with ear plugs and a considerable amount of pain. I started the second round of chemo right when I was starting to feel better. This time I was more prepared for the onslaught of the effects of the drug. I felt the now familiar symptoms crash through me again. The first round felt like a wave that crashes on an unsuspecting beachgoer who is tossed around in the surf. The second time felt like a smaller wave which came milliseconds after catching your breath from the initial wave. I had to fight to stand, coughing and spitting, struggling to find air. It was an exhausting feat.

I had been going to church with my family all fall. We were getting ready for Advent. Every year, St. Peter's Church holds a Lessons and Carols service. This service features the telling of the birth of Jesus plus selected Christmas carols. It's my favorite service of the Church year, as it combines beautiful sacred music with a soft, contemplative setting. This year would have more meaning, as the dark of winter seemed to envelop my whole mind and soul. Yet here was the spark of hope, light, and love that comes from a tiny child who will bring the end of suffering and death. Christmas was a glimmer of hope in my darkest time.

The church organist, Matt, started preparing the choir for the Lessons and Carols service. He teaches music education at a local preparatory school in Hamden in addition to leading the St. Peter's choirs. It turned out that Matt was a good friend of Dr. Baehring and had taught his daughter at Hamden Hall. Dr. Baehring's wife, Erikka, and daughter Katalina, both sang with the St. Peter's choir for Lessons and Carols this year. Over the few weeks of Advent, Caitlin and I were thrilled to sing and talk with Erikka, also a nurse practitioner, and Katalina, who was now studying at Northeastern University. Yet another coincidence.

The evening of the Lessons and Carols service, December 22nd, we happily sang in a beautiful and inspiring performance and worship service. Dr. Baehring and his son were in the congregation that night. We met briefly after the service. He was not in a lab coat, not at a computer screen, not wearing a stethoscope, not conducting neurological testing. He was another human being out with his son to hear his wife and daughter sing some beautiful music. Beyond my anger and pain, I found I saw Dr. Baehring in a new way that evening. He was just another medical professional treating other people, doing his best and supporting his family. This aspect of kinship brought a new hope to my treatment plan and was an added glimmer I needed that Christmas.

My second son, Vincent, turned one year old in the middle of December. In true Celella fashion, we had over 40 people come to our tiny house to celebrate his milestone. Although I had ear plugs in and barely ate, it was another time of hope. To see all the family, friends, and loved ones gathered together was almost overwhelming. The Christmas spirit continued to buoy my psyche.

I was filled with gratitude for all the people who had given me some hope with their gifts, well wishes, and prayers.

Christmas passed with the usual hustle and bustle. My brother and his family came up from Virginia and my in-laws came to stay with us again. I was feeling slightly better but still was in a cloud of anger, despair, and pain. Yes, there were some clear moments of hope, love, and peace, but I saw them only through a dark shroud.

Insurance Woes

Happy New Year! We all agreed that 2020 was going to be better than 2019. Things were going Ok until January 2nd, two days into the new year. I was getting ready for the same nonsense to get my Temozolomide ordered, processed, and shipped. I called Aetna Specialty Pharmacy and was told that the meds would be delivered on time, but first I needed to send in my co-pay. New year, new deductible. The nice lady on the phone hesitantly said, "Well, sir, it is a pretty high co-pay."

"Ok, how much?" I asked nonchalantly.

"The co-pay will be $3,553.94," she replied.

"Holy fucking shit?! Thirty-five hundred dollars!" I almost fell over.

"Um, $3,553.94, sir," she replied coldly.

"Jesus fucking Christ! It would probably be cheaper for my funeral!" My blood began to boil. My head increased its pounding.

"Oh, sir, please don't say that...."

"Oh, fuck off! You're not invited!" I interrupted her.

"I can offer you some resources for financial assistance."

"No, fuck that. I need these meds."

"I'm sorry, sir. I cannot send this medication without payment first."

"Jesus. Ok. I'll pay. I'm adding you to my haunt list."

I gave my credit card number and explained that she would be the second person I would haunt when I died. She seemed happy to rush through the rest of the transaction and get off the phone. I tried to calm down and not think of the huge amount of money I just put on my credit card. She told me, "Have a nice day." I told her, "Yeah, right. I'll see you in hell."

Later that afternoon, I received a termination letter from my employer, Hartford Healthcare. I knew this one was coming, but it was still a punch to the gut. I was to be transferred from short term disability (STD) payments to long term disability (LTD) payments through Prudential Insurance Company. Although this sounds absurd, it was necessary to be terminated from my duties at work to allow for the payments from Prudential and LTD and ensure that I would not get both a paycheck and LTD payment. Prudential was the company who managed my STD payments, and I was in close communication with my boss at Hartford Healthcare. I had known this was coming, but to actually receive the written notification of my termination was quite disheartening.

Prudential was quick to pick up my case and send 50% of my salary to me in monthly statements. Prudential did require that I apply for

Social Security benefits, as any benefit I received would be subtracted from my LTD check. I was horrified by this request. I thought that only old people, the horribly disabled, or scammers got Social Security checks. I reluctantly called the Social Security office. I thought I was in for something like a trip to the Department of Motor Vehicles (DMV). I thought of long lines, endless paperwork, bad service, and no benefit. I thought that I would be back to work by the time I even got any Social Security benefits.

Fortunately, I was very wrong. I called the office and they walked me through the entire application process. It took about 30 minutes on the phone and the people were so nice, thorough, and competent that it almost made my head spin. They got me a great wage, money for my children, and I was approved in only two days after applying. I am a true convert to government aid! It gave me the cash I needed to cover the next unanticipated hurdle.

What I did not anticipate was the need for COBRA coverage. The Consolidated Omnibus Budget Reconciliation Act (COBRA) allows for a limited period of health insurance coverage, usually at an increased rate. The rate of my COBRA plan was 102% of my actual cost, or $2,110.25 per month. That $2,110.25 would ensure that I could keep me and my family covered by health insurance. I could continue to pay ridiculously high co-pays for chemo drugs.

As the new year had commenced, I needed to again ask permission to see my doctors at YNHH. As a Hartford Healthcare employee, my Aetna insurance plan required that I only see Hartford

Healthcare providers (as Hartford Healthcare is a competitor of YNHH). However, in cases of emergency, Aetna will cover "out-of-network" costs. I didn't feel comfortable seeing a different provider while I was in the middle of cancer treatment.

I had to submit a document called a "Transition of Coverage," which would allow me to see my doctors at YNHH. I submitted the form about five times to five different numbers in the Aetna system. I later found that there had been a lapse of my insurance coverage because I had been terminated from Hartford Healthcare, and was not receiving benefits.

Another shocking letter came a few days later. This letter was from YNHH for services rendered on October 1st and November 1st, 2019 in the amount of $5,322.44. I had been charged for one radiation treatment in October (my last radiation session) in the amount of $2,581.12. Then I was charged $2,791.32 for the MRI in November. These two random bills were sent to me for collection because Aetna claimed they were "out-of-network."

In February 2019, my son Vincent had been admitted to YNHH, requiring a four-day ICU level of care. I was charged for his services at the out-of-network rate and met my out-of-pocket maximum deductible around that time. When I had the first seizure on June 20th, 2019, I went to YNHH, as it is closer to my house, was better equipped to treat my emergency, and my wife didn't want me to wake up to my co-workers at Midstate. From February 2019 to December 2019, I didn't pay a dime for two ambulance rides, two

ER visits, two hospitalizations, an awake craniotomy, two CT scans, five MRIs, a continuous EEG, numerous follow-up appointments, all the radiation sessions, all the chemo drugs, all the antiseizure drugs, and all the other miscellaneous services like blood work and professional fees. All of it probably totaled millions of dollars. All of it was covered under my Aetna policy. Except for the one session of radiation and one MRI. Even more infuriating was that other services, like blood work and the fees to Dr. Baehring, were covered.

I called Aetna to ask why these services were billed to me. They curtly answered that I was responsible for the charges and I should pay YNHH. I called Dr. Baehring's office, but there was little help. I then called Dr. Contessa's office. They looked into their records, and I got a personal phone call from Dr. Contessa to assure me that they had put the bills in just as they had for the other 32 sessions. They told me to call Aetna again. I made a verbal appeal to Aetna and explained the absurdity of charges. They told me they would get back to me in about a month. I told YNHH that I was in appeal with my insurance company and they put my case on hold.

A few weeks later, I received a letter from Aetna stating that my verbal appeal was denied on the grounds that the services rendered were still out-of-network. In the letter were instructions on second level appeal. I had to write a formal letter and include various sources that would support my claim. I called Dr. Baehring and Dr. Contessa and got letters written on my behalf. I painstakingly wrote a letter over the next week, something that would have taken me only an hour or two prior to the surgery. I was fortunate to have experience writing these letters and arguing a patient's case for an insurance company to cover services. As a hospitalist, at least once a week I would appeal, either verbally or written, to fight for coverage for the patients I was treating. Only now it took me much longer to write. A copy of the letter is below.

January 21, 2020
To: *Aetna Customer Resolution Team*
PO Box 14463
Lexington, KY 40512

From: *Joseph Andrew Celella*

Re: *Second-Level Appeal*

To whom it may concern:

This is a document to respond for a second level appeal. My name is Joseph Andrew Celella, Member number ▮▮▮▮▮▮▮*, Case ID:* ▮▮▮▮▮▮▮*.*

The dates below include an outstanding balance of $5322.44 payable to Yale New Haven Hospital (YNHH). The charges were sent to Aetna, however, they were denied. On December 9, 2019, I spoke with healthcare advocate Jesse at Aetna (ID number:

██████) *and gave my verbal appeal. I was notified on January 6, 2020 that the appeal had been denied. The denial reason was the network provider was out-of-network. I will refute this denial and will show why the above amount should be covered by Aetna.*

I am aware that my policy marks most Yale New Haven Hospital (YNHH)-affiliated providers out-of-network. However, my Aetna policy will cover out-of-network providers in cases of emergency. In February 2019, my son Vincent was admitted to YNHH requiring a four-day ICU level of care. I was charged for his services at the out-of-network rate and met my out-of-pocket maximum deductible around that time.

I had an emergency seizure on 6/20/2019 and the closest and best equipped hospital was Yale New Haven Hospital. Given that I had met my out-of-pocket maximum deductible for the year, my wife had the ambulance transport me to YNHH. Because my initial presentation was an emergency, the proceeding events of diagnosis of malignant brain tumor (anaplastic astrocytoma grade 3), seizure disorder, need for chemotherapy and therapeutic radiation were initiated. ***The costs of these proceeding events were all covered by my Aetna policy.***

On 6/25/2019, I underwent an awake craniotomy (brain surgery) to remove most of the 4 cm brain tumor. Over my hospital stay, I subsequently underwent a total of: one CT scan of the head, two brain MRIs, one functional brain MRI, and an additional MRI in the operating room while in surgery, all completed at YNHH. I was discharged from the hospital on 6/27/2019.

I had routine follow-up with Dr. Baehring on 7/8/2019. The biopsies showed the malignancy of my brain tumor. Chemotherapy and radiation were discussed and would commence six weeks following the initial surgery. Dr. Baehring managed the oral chemotherapy (Temozolomide (Temodar)). The schedule for the chemotherapy would be: initially 6 weeks Temodar taken every day, followed by six-28 day cycles starting on 11/13/2019 and ending around April of 2020.

I had routine follow up with Dr. Contessa on 7/11/2019. We discussed the initiation of radiation therapy. I was scheduled for an additional brain MRI and brain CT scan (completed on 7/25/2019) to pinpoint any residual malignant tumor cells and started on 33 sessions of radiation (sessions were daily Monday through Friday for 7 weeks). On 8/12/2019, therapeutic radiation and the initial six weeks of oral chemotherapy commenced.

Unfortunately, my course was complicated by rapid-onset of several grand mal seizures. On 8/26/2019, I was again admitted to YNHH with continuous seizure activity. I was placed on a continuous EEG monitoring system. I spent four days in the epilepsy unit. During the submission, I received an additional CT scan. My anti-seizure medications were adjusted and I was discharged on 8/31/2019.

After discharge, I continued on radiation and chemotherapy. I saw Dr. Baehring (or one of his physician assistants or APRNs) and Dr. Contessa weekly. I finished the initial 6 weeks of chemotherapy on 9/25/2019. **To reiterate, ALL of the above services rendered at YNHH were covered by my Aetna policy.**

I finished the radiation on 10/1/2019. This last day of radiation on 10/1/2019 is the first charge from YNHH. You will see on the reference below it is labeled "IMRT:CkV Visit at YM Therapeutic Radiology Smilow Cancer Hospital with Contessa, Joseph, MD from Oct 1, 2019 to Oct 31, 2019" in the amount of $2581.12. ***Each of the other 32 sessions of radiation were covered by my Aetna policy.*** *I also had a one month follow up with Dr. Contessa on 11/7/2019, which was also covered by Aetna.* ***In addition, every other visit with Dr. Contessa, all his colleagues, and every interaction with the Smilow Cancer/YNHH was covered by Aetna, despite Dr. Contessa being "out-of-network."***

I continued to see Dr. Baehring for additional courses of chemotherapy. I had an additional six- 28-day cycles to complete. As part of standard of care, Dr. Baehring ordered an MRI before starting the six rounds of chemotherapy. The MRI was to ensure no further disease progression had developed and to check the effectiveness of the therapeutic radiation. After reviewing the MRI on 11/1/2019, Dr Baehring determined I would start the chemotherapy cycles. I started the first cycle of Temozolomide (Temodar) on 11/13/2019.

The MRI that was scheduled on 11/1/2019 is the second charge from YNHH. You will see in the reference below it is labeled, "MRI BRAIN W WO IV CONTRAST Visit at MRI-Fitkin with Laurans, Monika S, PA on Nov 1, 2019" in the adjusted amount of $2791.32. To be clear, Monika Laurans PA is one of Dr Baehring's physician assistants. **This MRI was under doctor's orders and standard of care. Five previous MRIs (two MRIs prior to surgery, one functional MRI, one intraoperative MRI, and one prior to starting therapeutic radiation), were all covered by my Aetna policy.**

In summary, you can see the charges from YNHH seem to have been denied in error, given the same medically necessary care was ordered by the same physicians and covered under my Aetna policy. *In addition to the letter above, I have included the references for the two charges from YNHH (below) and a copy of the latest statement. I have also included letters from Dr. Baehring and Dr. Contessa to show the medical necessity for these MRIs and radiation.*

I hope this can shed some light on my frustration and the absurdity of the "out-of-network" denial I received from my Aetna policy. Please do not hesitate to contact me should you have any other questions or concerns.

Regards,

Joseph Andrew Celella APRN

I was very nervous to send the second-level appeal, as I anticipated three possible scenarios could result. Scenario one was Aetna agreeing with my appeal and then covering the expenses. This was the best-case scenario, and the one I hoped for. Scenario two was Aetna again refusing to pay, and I would end up with the $5,322.44 charge. In that case, I would start a third line appeal. The most terrifying, scenario three, was that Aetna would actually count all of the services I'd already had at YNHH as out-of-network, and then I would be responsible for covering literally hundreds of thousands of dollars.

Now add crippling anxiety from medical debt to my list of symptoms. This anxiety, and the fact that I was still trying to get the Transition of Coverage document submitted, made me take drastic steps to try and get as much care as I could in the Hartford Healthcare realm. I had blood work, an MRI in February, and other scattered tests completed at Hartford Healthcare facilities because of my fear of getting huge bills if I went to YNHH.

After a few weeks, I finally got the Transition of Coverage document submitted to the correct department and was approved. I was now able to see my physicians at YNHH and have my MRIs, blood work, and other tests completed at YNHH. I would still pay co-pays, but at least there was some coverage.

From a safety perspective, it is much better to keep all your tests and doctors in the same system. It allows for better continuity and better communication with the providers who are treating you. It was risky for me to have blood work and MRI tests performed in different systems. The MRI pictures done at Hartford Healthcare vary slightly and do not line up with the multiple other MRIs at YNHH. The electronic medical record (EMR) does not cross over to the Hartford Healthcare system unless I give a signed authorization. The blood work done at Hartford Healthcare used different reference ranges than the laboratories at YNHH. This could lead to unexpected results and could potentially lead to unnecessary and inappropriate changes to my medication. As an APRN, I was able to understand these nuances and anticipate problems while advocating for myself. The average patient does not have the skill or experience to anticipate these issues and advocate. This was all because I was essentially forced by my insurance company to receive tests at a different location, lest I receive a large bill.

Through February, I was calling Aetna every day to get information on my second line appeal. I was always given the same response, "The review team is working on it. We should have an answer by March. It maybe sooner, but we will let you know."

"Ok. Tell me your name again and a reference number for this call," I would respond. I have a notebook full of dates, times, names, and reference numbers of calls to Aetna, COBRA, and doctors' offices. I continued to press my case and noisily advocate for my appeal. Finally, on March 2nd, I got word that my appeal had been granted. I had won the fight. Thankfully, scenario one had occurred and Aetna covered the radiation therapy, while I covered a co-pay of $99.40.

Fortunately, I have the medical knowledge and expertise in filing appeals and coordinating my MRIs and blood work in a different hospital system. I know how to avoid medical errors while moving information across the different hospital systems. Part of my job as a hospitalist is advocating for and appealing to insurances for patients; I've gotten very good at it. I had to do it for myself, and I wonder about all the people that face such issues and don't know where to turn or whom to ask for help.

Despite all my gripes with my insurance company, I do have to thank them for all the coverage they provided. The tally of my premiums (about $10,000 per year for family coverage), plus the $6,000 deductible and the additional $3,000 out-of-pocket maximum, comes to a mere $19,000 yearly. This number pales in comparison to the probable one million dollars for all of my treatments and hospitalizations. Insurance is a necessary evil that was a huge part of saving my life. Although there are many aspects of insurance that seem asinine, I'm glad I had it.

I often think about the people I've treated that do not have health insurance. Patients for whom I was responsible for ordering tests, procedures, or other medical interventions that cost thousands of dollars. According to researchers from the New England Journal of Medicine, about 60% of personal bankruptcy is related to a medical cause. I've had patients who are more devastated that they are in the hospital than their actual medical condition. They have lost or cannot perform their jobs, cannot pay their bills, and wind up in serious debt or bankruptcy. Although there are social workers, resources, payment plans, and medication discounts, it is heart-wrenching to feel partially responsible for their plight. I want to scream, "All I wanted to do was to help! I wanted to heal the sick. I wanted to give comfort, peace, healing! Not bankrupt you!" Alas, this is the system in which we live here in America.

I am so lucky to have had savings, plus family and friends who offered financial support. Not having to worry about money was a burden lifted off my shoulders. I wish all my patients had the same support I had. I think there would be a lot of healthier people in this world.

Wednesday, January 8, 2020

Despite my looming battles with Aetna, I continued the drudgery of the chemo cycles. I started my third cycle on January 8th. After the New Year, I was feeling more energized and like a veteran of the chemo cycles. My head pounded, but I shrugged it off, thinking it would be there forever, so I might as well think of something else. My stomach ached, but I just went hungry. My ears rang and light pierced my eyes sharply, but I thought this was just the new normal. I pressed on like a marathon runner on mile 13.1—halfway there.

I dealt with the insurance appeals and started to work on adjusting to what I thought was my new normal. I started reading more medical journals. I wrote hundreds of pages of words I couldn't read. I wrote until my hand was stiff, the pen ran out of ink, and I could finally read the words I had written. I was still working on continuing medical education (CME) credits, a large part of renewing my board certification, which was set to expire in July of 2020.

I started running again. I had run five miles the morning that I had the first seizure, June 20, 2019. I had been a marathon runner, but since grad school, having kids, drinking too much beer, and a general lack of hustle, I had gotten out of shape. I was starting to increase my running in the fall of 2018 and gradually increased my distance. By June 2019, I was running three to five miles about three times a week. Then POW! Brain cancer and surgery.

I finally dug out my running shoes and went for a jog in January, weighing about 40 pounds less than last year. I went two miles that first day in late January. It was an abnormally warm winter, so I would bundle up and pound the pavement as long as it was at least 20°F.

I felt free. The pain in my head subsided when I ran, and I could focus. Runner's high coursed through my veins like heroin. The next day, I ran four miles. Since I had lost 40 pounds, I immediately started running faster and stronger than I had in June. Five miles two days later. I finished out January having clocked a couple dozen miles in two weeks.

Wednesday, February 5, 2020

I met with one of Dr. Baehring's PAs in early February. I was still slightly immunosuppressed, but able to start cycle number four on February 5th. I had the same familiar symptoms for the first week, but then they waned quite fast. I was feeling better by the end of day 10, less than a week after finishing the five-day cycle of pills. I kept up with running and was getting stronger every day. I kept losing weight, but mostly from running, not from eating less.

I was still singing with the Camerata and my church choir. These two communities were cheering me on as I progressed through the cycles of chemo. I was so fortunate to have such a wide base of support. No one can fight this battle alone. I had people checking in on me and my family every step of the way.

I continued to keep myself busy, studying medicine and completing CMEs. By the end of the month, I had submitted all the necessary paperwork to process a renewal of my APRN board certification. I was starting to read and write to about 85% of what I had been doing before the brain surgery and seizures. While I was taking the chemo, I experienced a noticeable decrease in my ability to read, write, and speak. However, a few days after finishing the Temozolomide, my concentration, reading, and writing would return to almost normal, only to be battered again as the next cycle started.

As part of my "physical therapy" to re-teach my brain to remember words and write correctly, I started to write this memoir. I would wait to put the kids down to sleep at 7 PM, then get a small cup of coffee and plow through a few hours of writing. I was able to give myself an increased challenge by writing at the end of the day. It was always harder to think, comprehend, and work later at night.

The first week was very difficult, with lots of missing words, misspelling almost every other word, and often losing my train of thought. Gradually, I got faster. I didn't need the coffee anymore. I had notebooks of words I had misspelled, but now I was remembering those words and spelling them correctly. I was churning out about 2,500 words every two-and-a-half hours.

I also continued to paint. I was commissioned by my parents to paint their bedroom. The cape-style house made the bedroom a labyrinth of angles and tight spaces. It took me a week of six-hour days to complete the room. I find painting oddly therapeutic and would often listen to audiobooks or let my mind wander while listening to music. I got into audiobooks while making the 45-minute commute to grad school at Yale's West Campus in Orange, Connecticut. After I lost my ability to read, audiobooks were a way to continue that familiar hobby.

When listening to audiobooks, I was able to turn up the speed of the readers to about two times the normal rate. A 12-hour book became a six-hour book, which I could finish in about three days. I started on a journey to "read" the entire New International Version (NIV) Bible—80 hours of audiobook, but only 40 hours with the faster reading setting.

While painting, I plowed through the first five books: Genesis, Exodus, Leviticus, Numbers, and Deuteronomy in one day. Paint spackled the walls as I heard the tales of creation, Abraham, Isaac, Jacob, Noah, Joshua, King Saul, and King David. I was enraptured again by the prophecies and works of Elijah, Isaiah, Daniel, Samson, Job, and Jeremiah. I moved into the New Testament, with the stories of Jesus and his disciples, which culminated with the dramatic chapter of Revelation. I finished the entire Bible in a little less than six weeks.

Being a preacher's kid, my parents having met in Divinity School, I was well-versed in the Bible. I was baptized, married, and then had both of my sons baptized at the same quaint Episcopal church, St. Peter's. Caitlin (also a preacher's kid, her father an Episcopal priest), also had a long history at St. Peter's. We continued our life in faith with that wonderful community. It was like having a whole second family. While there were disagreements and mishaps, there was an abundance of kindness, respect for different beliefs, a sense of belonging, and most importantly, love.

This small yet vibrant community was with me, Caitlin, and my children from earlier and happier times, all the way to the initial shock of the cancer diagnosis, the seizures, and every chemo and radiation treatment. They offered support with wisdom, comforting prayer, and abundant food. In reading the Bible, the people of St. Peter's exemplified what it meant to be followers of Christ. We are eternally grateful.

I had a meeting scheduled with my oncologist at the end of February, per the normal treatment course. Prior to meeting with Dr. Baehring, I noticed my Keppra was running low. I called the pharmacy and quickly realized the incorrect number of pills had been dispensed after an incorrect order was placed by one of the PAs.

I was taking 2000 milligrams of Keppra twice a day. Keppra comes in 1000 mg tablets, so I would take two tablets (to make 2000 mg) in the morning and two tablets at night. My Aetna insurance requested that I have 90-day supplies of this drug. Two tablets twice a day is four tablets a day; four times 90 days is 360 tablets. In January, I was given 180 tablets, only half the supply I needed. By the middle of February, about 45 days' worth of pills, I was coming to the end of my supply.

I called Aetna and my pharmacy and asked for refills, but because of my insurance company's 90-day supply rule, Aetna would not authorize another refill on day 45. I remember one conversation I'd had with an Aetna representative when I'd asked, "Would you like to pay for $500 of Keppra, or would you like me to have more seizures? Then you'd be on the hook for about $500,000 for an emergency hospital stay."

"I see your point, sir," was the response.

After additional phone calls to the pharmacy, Dr. Baehring's office, and Aetna, I finally got the additional Keppra pills—for a nominal fee of $487.95.

This is a classic example of what the healthcare system calls the Swiss cheese model. Essentially, there are many safeguards to prevent errors in healthcare; however, there may be little holes in each safeguard. If the holes align, it's like a block of Swiss cheese where you can see through the multiple holes, and harm can come to a patient. In my case, the initial order by the PA was placed incorrectly: 1000 mg of Keppra (one pill) twice a day rather than 2000 mg (two pills) twice a day. Then the pharmacist didn't see the dosage change (from 2000 mg to 1000 mg). Finally, I didn't notice the incorrect count of the meds until I was almost out of them. Several breaks in the system, like a holey block of Swiss cheese, could have caused me to have a seizure before receiving the pills I needed.

This happens all the time in medicine. Dosages are missed, drugs are given incorrectly, and people get hurt or die. There is a well-known study published in 1999 called "To Err is Human." It became a book, reviewed every few years, and is widely circulated between medical providers. According to a 2016 Johns Hopkins' study, medical errors account for 250,000 American deaths per year. That's the equivalent of close to TWO Boeing 747 airplanes killing everyone on board EVERY DAY.

Later that month, Dr. Baehring and I sat in his office with two residents and one medical student. I stood on my soapbox and explained my frustration about the medication error. Turning to the residents and medical students, I said, "Don't let this happen to you—both the medical error and cancer." They let out a shy laugh. I hope it made an impression, but they probably have forgotten.

Friday, March 6, 2020

Time marched on, day by day. I kept running, tallying 80 miles during the month of March. We continued singing at church and now had nicer news to report to our fellow parishioners. I was feeling better and better. I had my usual blood draw and started to get ready for my next chemo cycle.

Prior to starting this regimen, I was found to have a low platelet count. Platelets are part of the blood that help it to clot. If your platelet count is too low, you are more prone to hemorrhage or bleeding. The chemotherapy affects the fast-growing cells in your body (i.e., tumor cells or immune cells), and it can also affect platelets. They don't generate as quickly as they should. The medical term for this is thrombocytopenia, and it is a well-known adverse effect of chemotherapy. Fortunately, I had no complications of bleeding, but did have a delayed start to chemo cycle number five.

The usual effects of chemo waned in a few days. I was feeling strong, like I was ready to get back to work. I began the process to restart my credentialing and get rehired at Hartford Healthcare. The credentialing process usually takes about two to three months. The credentialing application consists (partially) of: my education diplomas, APRN and RN licensure information, malpractice insurance, background checks, applications to bill insurance companies, National Provider Identifier (NPI) number, DEA license certificate, controlled substance license, Advanced Cardiac Life

Support (ACLS) certification, continuing education certificates, and any other special licenses. This exhaustive list is checked, cross examined, then submitted to a number of professional organizations and insurance companies. The information is gathered to ensure that I am who I say I am, and to confirm that I am certified and licensed to practice medicine.

While waiting for this process to be completed, I kept reading and writing, getting close to the sixth and final cycle of chemotherapy. Then the novel COVID-19, or Coronavirus, swept through the USA with blistering force. I read a New York Times abstract of a mysterious virus in China in early February, and scoffed at the prediction of a pandemic. I thought about some of the epidemics which have swept through during my career, such as bird flu (Avian Flu-H5N1 in 2004, 2014), swine flu (H1N1 in 2009), SARS (2002), MERS (2012), Ebola (2013-2015), and Zika virus (2015). I thought nothing of this new virus.

Boy, was I wrong. By the middle of March, schools had been canceled, isolation orders placed, and lots of people were dying. Selfishly, I was not happy to go into isolation. I felt I'd been in isolation over the last eight months dealing with brain cancer. Now I wanted to get back to work. As a critical care and ICU-trained APRN, I felt like I should be on the front lines. It was as if my team was at the Superbowl and I was on the sidelines. I felt like I was letting people down. But I was in the high-risk group, immunosuppressed on chemo, so I wouldn't be much help if I got sick and took up an ICU bed or a funeral parlor. My family and I were reluctantly isolated.

I had a few surgical masks around the house which I had gathered from various hospitals over the years. I went to the grocery store once a week. No singing, no church, no socialization. Only running. Again, I was stripped of my coping mechanisms.

I got blood work done off-site and did not go to YNHH. I had virtual appointments with Dr. Baehring. My platelets were good and I had enough immunity to start up cycle number six.

Friday, April 3, 2020

I started my last round of chemo during the third week of isolation and lockdown. I finished the cycle and was back to normal within two days. I felt indestructible, but apprehensive about getting back to work. I felt guilty for not being able to work in the hospital, and anxiously read all the literature I could about the COVID-19 virus. I followed along as the guidelines changed by the minute. I asked friends and colleagues who were working in the ICUs how bad it was. How many cases? How did it feel?

I wanted in! I wanted to help and fight as I was trained to do. Most people I talked to told me to stay at home as long as I could. They said not to come back until COVID had gone away, but I was both arrogant and determined to press on and start as soon as I could. I would get an MRI to document progression/curation of the astrocytoma on April 23rd and I would have blood work the next day to ensure my immune system was working. Last was a meeting with Dr. Baehring on the 27th, and if all clear, I could go back to work Saturday, May 2nd.

While I was anxiously waiting, I got a call from a friend at church who is an anesthesiologist. Anesthesiologists are doctors whose primary function is managing patients in ORs. They use medications to sedate, intubate, maintain sedation through a surgery, and then extubate patients after the surgical procedure. Another critical function is to intubate patients who cannot breathe or manage their own airways. To intubate someone, the anesthesiologist uses a dull blade to force the tongue downward, expose the opening to the windpipe or trachea, insert a tube into the trachea, then connect the tube to a ventilator machine. If you have never seen this procedure— and are not squeamish—you can watch thousands of videos on YouTube. It is truly a barbaric procedure with lots of sputum, drool, and sometimes blood.

When COVID hit southern New England, the hospitals did not have enough of the personal protective equipment (PPE) that anesthesiologists require to intubate someone, such as masks and face shields. The community had to help make these items so the anesthesiologists would be safe and patients could be properly treated. My church family at St. Peter's, along with my wife and I, found a way to make Tyvek hoods that would shield the hospital staff. Like Rosie the Riveter, I set to work and made about 45 of these hoods. If I couldn't be on the front lines, I would damn well be in the supply chain by making PPE.

On Thursday the 27th, I went for the MRI. Everything was on lockdown because of COVID precautions. Masks were required. In the cramped space of the MRI machine, I could feel the stink of my bad breath against the fabric of the mask. I was stricken by claustrophobia, and breathed the stale air even faster. I used my chin to loosen the mask and push it down my face and onto my chin so I could get some fresh air and make it through the test.

I had asked for a disc to review the images, but unfortunately the CD burner wasn't working. It was late in the day, and I had to come back the following day to get blood drawn. I felt discouraged that I wouldn't be able to see the scans and know if any progress had been made.

The next morning, I went back to the clinic to have my blood drawn for routine monitoring. This was day 21 of the last cycle, and it was important to show that I was not immunosuppressed and could return to work. After the needle stick, I went to the MRI department and asked for a CD of my MRI. I was told that the CD burner was still not working and I couldn't have a disc.

"I'm not leaving this office until I have a disc in my hand," I firmly told the MRI technician. After my steadfast denial to leave and multiple phone calls by the technicians, about an hour later, I finally had the disc.

Loading the images onto the computer as soon as I got home, I saw that they looked really good. Less areas of FLAIR (brain lesion), and no evidence of any increase in cancer. Although I didn't have the official report, and I wouldn't meet Dr. Baehring until Monday, I felt pretty good.

Monday I had a virtual meeting with Dr. Baehring because of COVID restrictions. Through his staid German affect, he greeted me with a warm smile. He showed me the results of the MRI and explained that there was no further evidence of cancer progression. I briefly asked how his family was doing, and we chatted as if we were colleagues rather than doctor and patient. We set up the next

MRI to be completed in July. I profusely thanked him for all he and his staff at YNHH had done for me. I am eternally grateful for all their work to keep me alive and safe.

With my suspicions confirmed—no further cancer in my brain—my family and I were thrilled. The surgery, chemo, and radiation had worked to give me essentially a clean bill of health. We made several ecstatic phone calls to family and friends. I felt like I had just crossed the 26.2-mile line at the end of the marathon. Now I was gearing up to get back to work. My reading, writing, and speech were normal, and because of my diet and exercise routines, I was healthier than ever.

Saturday, May 2, 2020

In the middle of a global pandemic, I crossed the threshold of Midstate Medical Center and returned to work. The battle against COVID-19 had waned a bit. I felt like I was stepping onto the beaches of Normandy, but three months after the initial fighting had begun. The staff bore battle scars. There was still fear in the eyes of the doctors and nurses. But hope was also abundant. There were signs of decreasing COVID cases, with more people being treated and released, and a lower death toll. I hope I gave some renewed hope as a fresh member of the team.

My boss and Midstate were committed to making my return a successful and safe one. The first few days at work, I saw only three patients. This was a far cry from the usual 15-20 patients per day before I left almost a year earlier. In a convenient turn, two of the three patients I had seen a year before. I was able to access my notes and re-read some of my interactions from over a year prior. I finished rounding with the three patients, wrote my notes, and spoke to a bunch of doctors and nurses who had supported me during my 11 months of absence. It was so good to see everyone—albeit behind masks—and it gave a renewed sense of fulfillment to my vocational life.

Over the next few weeks of work, I found myself getting back to my usual routines. I was able to keep up with my old pace of seeing patients, reviewing charts, writing notes, and admitting and discharging patients. I gradually increased my work flow to the usual 15-20 patients. It felt so good to be on the other side of the bed, treating patients rather than being one myself.

I found that I had a dramatic shift in my perspective while seeing patients. I could empathize with patients on a deeper level. Whether I was delivering good news or bad, I could relate. I had a young, 22-year-old female admitted with chest pain and shortness of breath. She had a blood test that showed she may have had a blood clot in her lungs. I ordered a CT scan of her chest. I did not find a blood clot, but I did find a 3.5 cm thymus tumor in the middle of her chest. While explaining the results to her, I couldn't help but think of my own 3.6 cm brain tumor and how it felt to be told such devastating news.

I also examined a 53-year-old female who wanted to get out of the hospital faster than was safe. She had been admitted with an asthma exacerbation, requiring steroids and oxygen. She could barely walk a few feet without gasping for air. I was reminded of my own struggles—wanting to leave the hospital after having multiple seizures, still not able to speak, and having multiple mini seizures.

I had an 87-year-old man who was admitted because he'd had an episode of slurred speech, which often points to a stroke. All the usual tests for strokes were completed and there was no evidence that he had suffered a stroke. I brought the good news to the man and his family. "I'm happy to tell you that you did not have a stroke. All your tests look good, and you can go home." Such joy and elation. The man and his family thanked me profusely. The well of pride and accomplishment in discharging him was reminiscent of hearing my news of no further evidence of cancer in my brain.

Going room to room delivering good news, bad news, updates, and treatment options can vary widely depending on the patient's particular medical issue. Arranging life-saving surgery, discharging a healed patient, or placing a patient on hospice and then signing their death certificate can all be done within any given hour throughout my day. With my newfound patient perspective, I identified more closely and empathized with patients and their families. I had experienced life, death, health, and malaise both as a medical practitioner and a patient while gaining a profound acceptance of my own mortality.

The Future

This profound experience has highlighted a deeper understanding of the human condition. Through my faith, I have found the wonders of the divine. After the brain surgery, I did not gain any superpowers, but I did experience an odd feeling of seeing people in a way which they all seem familiar. I took this as a revelation of our inherent divinity. Everything that lives is connected to others as created beings. I find myself trying to ensure continued life to all creatures. I avoid driving over squirrels that bound across the road. I do not squash bugs or spiders, although I do make exceptions for mosquitoes and ticks. I try to find the divine life in all creatures.

I have profound regret for all the people I abused over the phone. I have come close to death, and often think of my own mortality, and how I want to live as long as I can—to be with my family, friends, and to offer my service to those who are sick and hospitalized. I think of the Golden Rule, to treat others as you want to be treated. This rule, found in almost every major world religion, ancient mysticism, and even political systems, ought to be the cornerstone of living a good life.

Although I think of it in a religious framework, this idea of interconnectivity and treating others as divine could be thought of from a scientific viewpoint. Take the Law of Conservation of Matter, which states matter cannot be created nor destroyed; it only changes form. If an ice cube is heated, it will cease to be an ice cube, but becomes liquid water. Heat the water further, and it will cease to be water, changing form to become vapor. The same goes for the Law of Entropy or the Second Law of Thermodynamics, which states that in a closed system, the total entropy will never decrease. However, in the universe, we see that entropy will always strive for equilibrium. An ice cube will always eventually end up at the same temperature as the ambient room. If placed in a 70°F room, the ice cube will melt to become 70°F liquid water. It will not be destroyed, nor created; it has only changed form.

When we think about human life, it can be simply like an ice cube which changes form to become liquid water. We are all made of the same atoms and molecules that make up everything in the universe. These atoms and molecules coalesce to make cells, blood, heart, lung, brain, hormones, and organic mechanisms that support life. These atoms can be traced back to the beginning of the universe and the Big Bang. They have been changing form to make the building blocks of planet Earth. They make up the core, mantle, and volcanos. They change form to build rocks, trees, and water. They rearrange to give rise to organic compounds—to build dinosaurs, bugs, whales, and everyone you have heard about through history and beyond. The atoms inside you, making up the various parts of your organs, bacteria, and even allowing you to read these words, may have been part of mountain building, ocean forming, or star creation. It is a truly divine thought that we are made from the same material as stars.

This divinity of humankind challenges me to treat everyone I meet with the same awe and respect that any divine being ought to be given. We all have pieces of eternity and divinity within our being. This idea has resonated with me since singing the Ralph Vaughan Williams piece with Walt Whitman's poem, *"For my enemy is dead—a man divine as myself is dead."* When pronouncing a patient dead, I think of this phrase. Obviously, my patients are not my enemy. The Whitman poem is about him treating an enemy confederate soldier in the Civil War. But my patient, a human— divine as myself—is dead, has some extraordinary consequences. I utter a solemn, "May light perpetual shine upon them," and think of their body, soul, and being changing form, their atoms rearranged, creating something new and divine.

So what is next for me? I am cured of brain cancer. I have run the marathon and finished spectacularly well. Now I have constant vigilance. I have changed my diet radically to eat healthier. I do not drink alcohol to help avoid seizures. Obviously, I do not smoke cigarettes, because they cause cancer. I do not smoke cannabis to not only avoid any altered state so I can monitor for seizures, but also obviously because I cannot be impaired while handling my patients' lives. I run many miles every week to stay strong and physically fit. I continue to sing and seek out evidence of God. I am trying to pay back student loans and set my family up for financial security when I perish. I cherish every moment I am on this Earth. I mourn the patients who I've seen pass away, and the people who have succumbed to cancer and other diseases. I look for opportunities to continue to help heal the sick and bring "Better health for all people," which is the Yale School of Nursing mission statement.

In my office, I have displayed a Ralph Waldo Emerson poem that reads,

"What is success?

To laugh often and much;

to win the respect of intelligent people
and the affection of children;

to earn the appreciation of honest critics
and endure the betrayal of false friends;

to appreciate the beauty;

to find the best in others;

to leave the world a bit better, whether
by a healthy child, a garden patch
or a redeemed social condition;

to know even one life has breathed
easier because you have lived.

This is to have succeeded!"

As I finish these pages, I stop to look at that quote. I realize that I have been blessed to have met every condition for success. I hope that my children and family, my patients, and everyone—all as divine as I am—can say the same.

Editor's Note

Andy wrote "I have run the marathon and finished spectacularly well." That's the truth. He loved all of us without measure and never stopped working to make sure he took care of everyone he laid eyes on.

After two cancer recurrences and successful surgeries two and three, Andy decided in April 2023 not to go under the knife for a fourth time. He was laughing, driving, felling trees in the backyard, and playing soccer with our boys right until he made the decision to enter hospice.

Typical Andy: he entertained everyone during their visits, describing his gratitude for love and a life well lived. He continued to thank the staff and his doctors, and to manage his own care. He scooted over so I could snuggle him in bed, ate all of Nonni's food, wheeled himself out to the back lawn for fresh air, and perked right up when the boys came to spend time with him.

He was communicative and loving until his last breath, and is remembered and missed every day.

-Caitlin Celella, Andy's wife

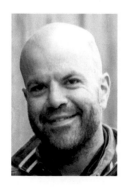

Joseph Andrew Celella

August 4, 1987-June 10, 2023

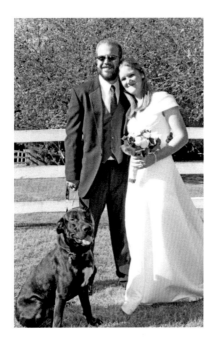

Andy and Caitlin at their wedding reception
joined by Angus, Cheshire, CT, October 8, 2011

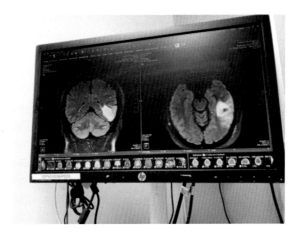

Andy's pre-op MRI images, June 21, 2019

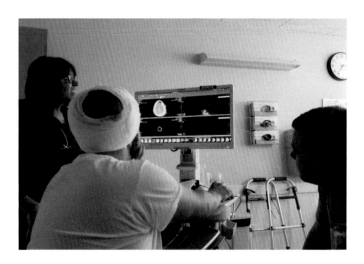

Andy reviewing his scans and chart with his team
while recovering from surgery, June 26, 2019

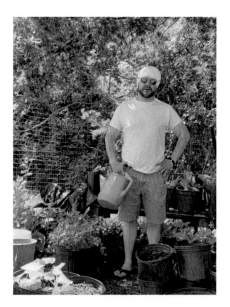

Post-op day 3 and working in Nonni's garden, June 28, 2019

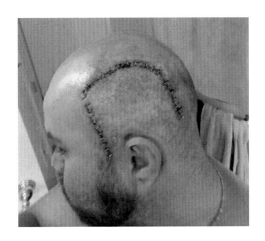

Surgical site before staple removal, July 2019

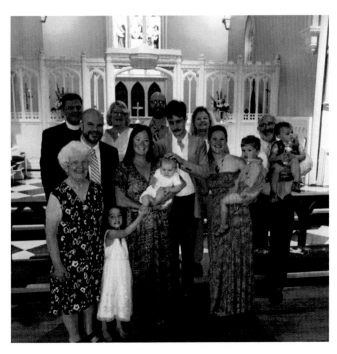

Vinny's baptism, St. Peter's Episcopal Church, Cheshire, CT, June 30, 2019

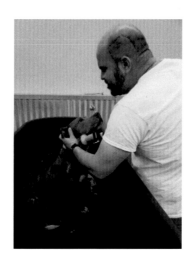

Andy and Whit, August 2019

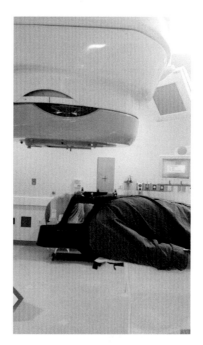

Andy ready for radiation—in his mask and on the table,
September 2019

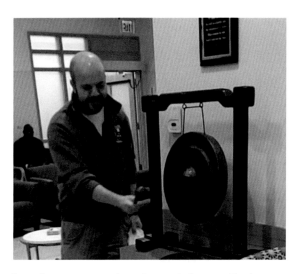

Ringing the gong to signal surviving radiation treatments,
October 1, 2019

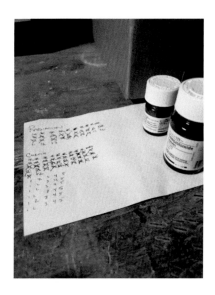

Andy's radiation and chemotherapy countdown (left),
with bottles of chemotherapy pills (right), September 2019

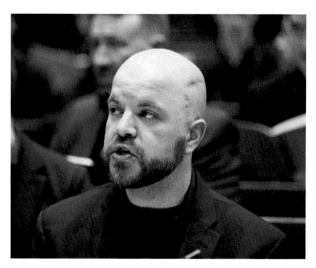

Singing with Yale Camerata, Fall 2019

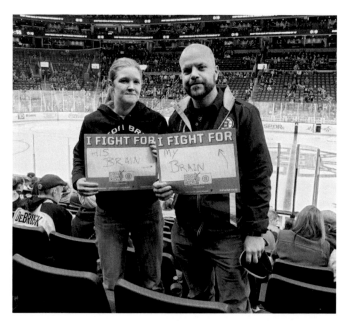

Andy and Caitlin at the Bruins' "Hockey Fights Cancer" game,
October 29, 2019

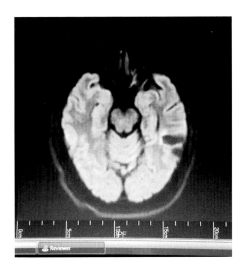

MRI of Andy's brain after radiation and chemo; looking good, so back to work! April 3, 2020

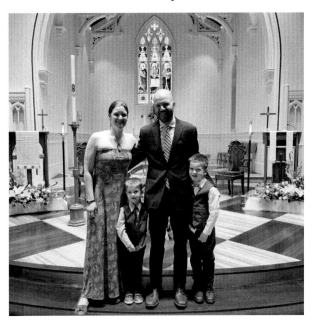

Andy, Caitlin, Ralphie, and Vinny at Easter, St. Peter's Church, Cheshire, CT, April 2023

Further reading

Awake craniotomy

https://thejns.org/focus/view/journals/neurosurg-focus/18/4/foc.2005.18.4.6.xml

https://www.ncbi.nlm.nih.gov/pmc/articles/PMC4710339/#ref2

https://journals.lww.com/rca/Fulltext/2018/06002/Awake_cranioto my__indications,_benefits,_and.9.aspx

https://www.uptodate.com/contents/anesthesia-for-awake-craniotomy

Glioma

https://www.uptodate.com/contents/clinical-presentation-diagnosis-and-initial-surgical-management-of-high-grade-gliomas?search=awake%20craniotomy&source=search_result&sel ectedTitle=3~10&usage_type=default&display_rank=3

https://www.uptodate.com/contents/classification-and-pathologic-diagnosis-of-gliomas?search=astrocytoma&source=search_result&selectedTitle =1~73&usage_type=default&display_rank=1

Medical bankruptcy

https://www.ncbi.nlm.nih.gov/pmc/articles/PMC5865642/

https://www.nejm.org/doi/full/10.1056/NEJMp1716604?url_ver=Z
39.88-2003rfr_id=ori:rid:crossref.org&rfr_dat=cr_pub%3dpubmed

References

https://www.youtube.com/watch?v=XHTtQ9b3heQ
-Cow video, "Cows jump over a white line while crossing the road"

https://www.youtube.com/watch?v=BoXXJpawB_M&t=16s
-Andy's awake craniotomy on Fox61 News, "This man is awake, and singing, during brain surgery"